Cardiovascular Care

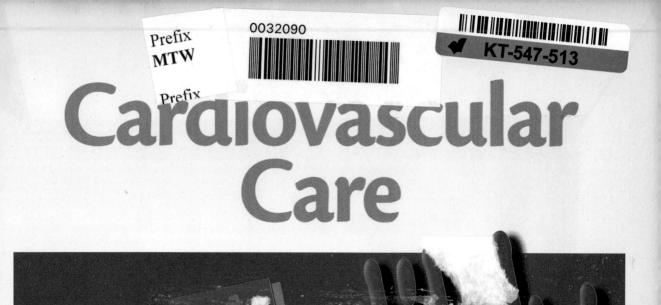

made Incredibly Visual!™

Lippincott Williams & Wilkins
a Wolters Kluwer business
Philadelphia · Baltimore · New York · London
Buenos Aires · Hong Kong · Sydney · Tokyo

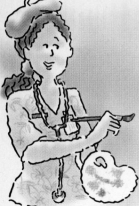

Staff

Executive Publisher
Judith A. Schilling McCann, RN, MSN

Editorial Director
David Moreau

Clinical Director
Joan M. Robinson, RN, MSN

Senior Art Director
Arlene Putterman

Art Director
Mary Ludwicki

Senior Managing Editor
Jaime Stockslager Buss, ELS

Clinical Project Manager
Carol A. Saunderson, RN, BA, BS

Editors
Brenna H. Mayer, Nancy Priff, Liz Schaeffer,
Gale Thompson, Libby Tucker, Susan Williams

Copy Editors
Kimberly Bilotta (supervisor), Scotti Cohn,
Karen C. Comerford, Amy Furman,
Shana Harrington, Pamela Wingrod

Designers
Marsha Biderman, Lynn Foulk

Illustrators
Bot Roda, Betty Winnberg, Jacqueline Facciolo,
Joseph John Clark, Judy Newhouse,
Leah Rhoades Purvis, Donna S. Morris

Digital Composition Services
Diane Paluba (manager), Joyce Rossi Biletz

Associate Manufacturing Manager
Beth J. Welsh

Editorial Assistants
Megan L. Aldinger, Karen J. Kirk, Linda K. Ruhf

Design Assistants
Georg W. Purvis IV, Eoanna Larsen

Indexer
Barbara Hodgson

CARIV010606—021006

Library of Congress Cataloging-in-Publication Data

Cardiovascular care made incredibly visual.
   p. ; cm.
   Includes bibliographical references and index.
1. Heart—Diseases — Nursing — Handbooks, manuals, etc. 2. Critical care medicine — Handbooks, manuals, etc. 3. Heart — Diseases — Nursing — Atlases. 4. Critical care medicine — Atlases. I. Lippincott Williams & Wilkins.
[DNLM: 1. Cardiovascular Diseases — nursing — Atlases. 2. Cardiovascular Diseases — nursing — Handbooks. WY 49 C267 2007]
RC674.C3588 2007
616.1'2025—dc22
ISBN 13 978-1-58255-636-9
ISBN 10 58255-636-9 (alk. paper)   200600471

Contents

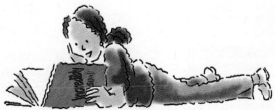

AT THE MOVIES

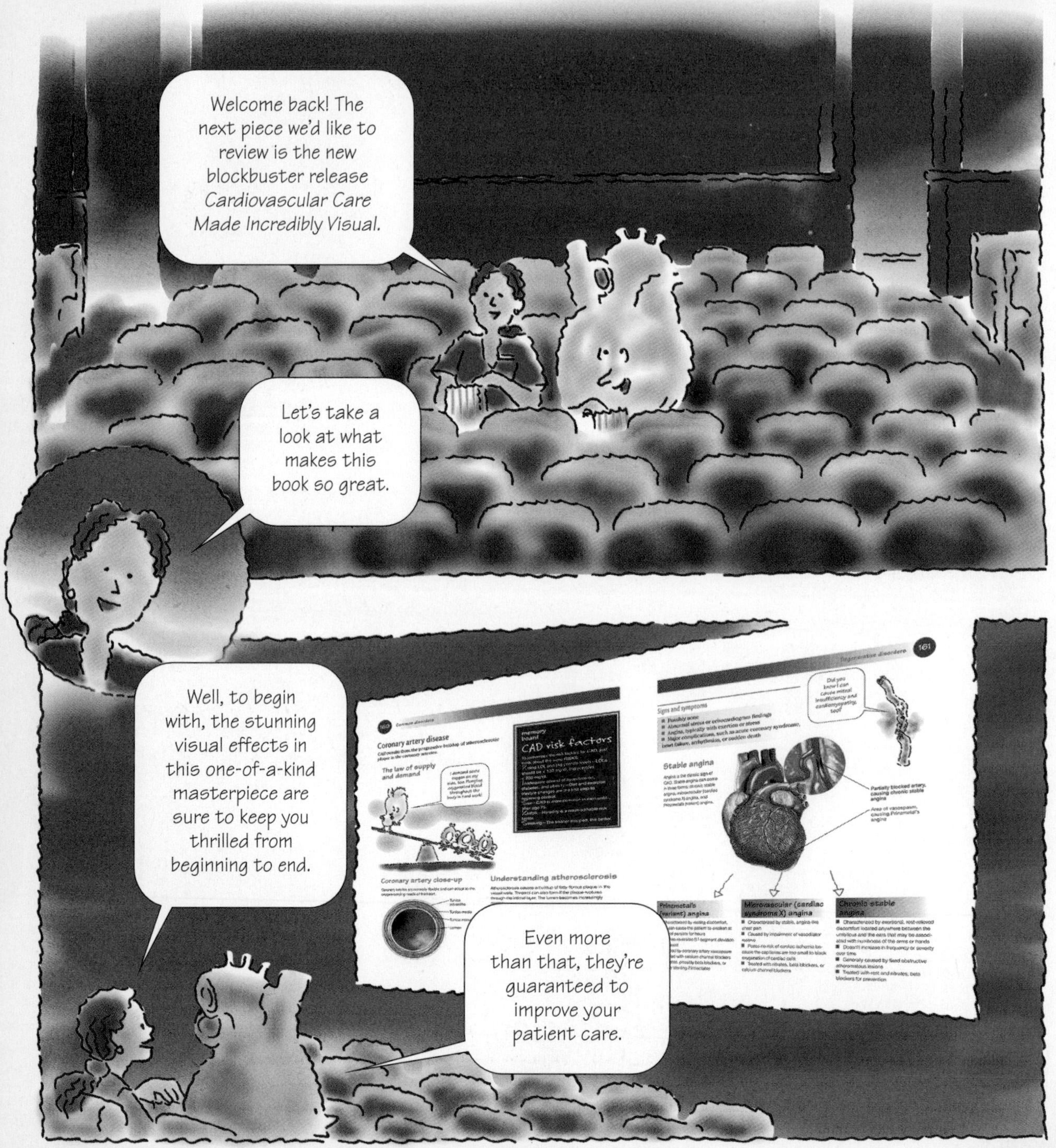

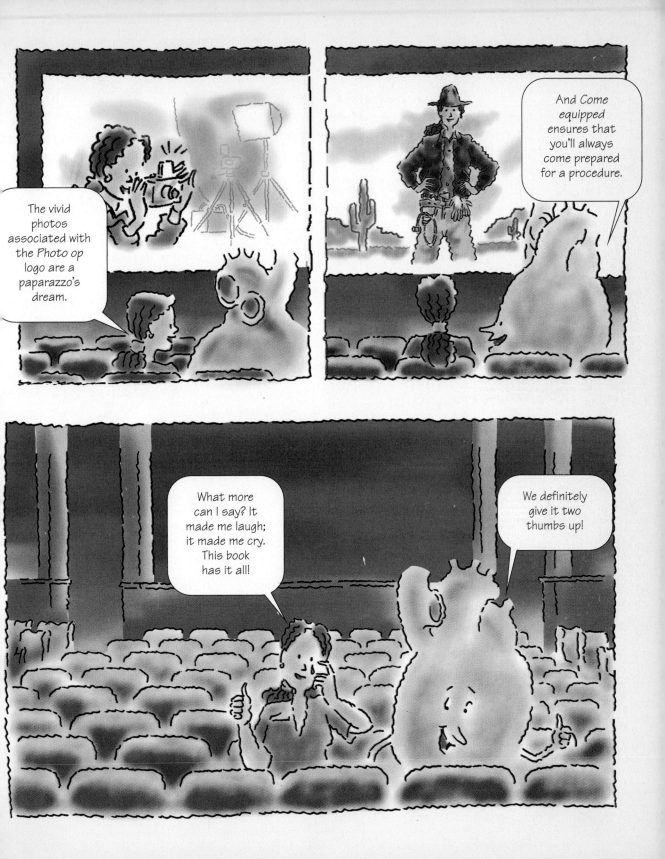

Contributors and consultants

Diane M. Allen, ANP, BC, MSN
Cardiovascular Nurse Practitioner
Womack Army Medical Center
Fort Bragg, N.C.

Deborah M. Berry, RN, MSN
Internal Consultant, Resource Management
MedStar Health
Lutherville, Md.

Louise M. Diehl-Oplinger, RN, MSN, CCRN, APRN-BC
Advanced Practice Nurse
Coventry Cardiology Associates
Phillipsburg, N.J.

Thomas L. Petricini, RN, MSN
Nursing Educator
Sharon (Pa.) Regional Health System
School of Nursing

Amy Shay, RN, MS, CCRN, CNS
Pulmonary Clinical Nurse Specialist
Miami Valley Hospital
Dayton, Ohio

Sharon Wing, RN, MSN
Associate Professor
Cleveland State University

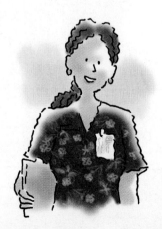

1 Anatomy and physiology

Scene 1, take 1. Anatomy and physiology is at the heart of cardiovascular care.

Location of the heart

The heart lies beneath the sternum within the mediastinum, a cavity that contains the tissues and organs separating the two pleural sacs. In most people, two-thirds of the heart extends to the left of the body's midline, close to the left midclavicular line. The heart rests obliquely so that its broad part, the base, is at its upper right and the pointed end, the apex, is at its lower left. The apex is the point of maximal impulse, where heart sounds are loudest.

> Sure I lean to the left, but I'm really politically neutral.

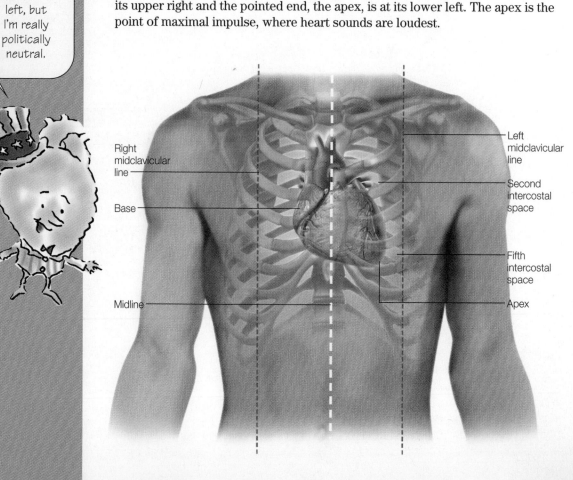

Right midclavicular line

Base

Midline

Left midclavicular line

Second intercostal space

Fifth intercostal space

Apex

Structures of the heart

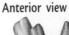

Heart wall layers

■ The *epicardium*, the outer layer, is made up of squamous epithelial cells overlying connective tissue.

■ The *myocardium*, the middle layer, forms most of the heart wall. It has striated muscle fibers that cause the heart to contract.

■ The *endocardium*, the heart's inner layer, consists of endothelial tissue with small blood vessels and bundles of smooth muscle.

Pericardium
Fibrous pericardium
Serous pericardium
(parietal layer)

Serous pericardium
(visceral layer [epicardium])

Myocardium (muscle layer)

Endocardium

Anterior view

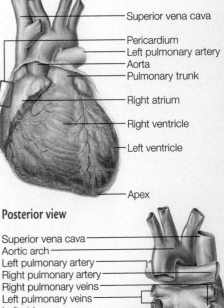

Superior vena cava

Pericardium
Left pulmonary artery
Aorta
Pulmonary trunk

Right atrium

Right ventricle

Left ventricle

Apex

Posterior view

Superior vena cava
Aortic arch
Left pulmonary artery
Right pulmonary artery
Right pulmonary veins
Left pulmonary veins
Left atrium
Right atrium
Inferior vena cava

Right ventricle
Left ventricle

A sac called the *pericardium* surrounds the heart and roots of the great vessels. It consists of two layers: the fibrous pericardium (tough, white fibrous tissue) and serous pericardium (thin, smooth inner portion). The serous pericardium also has two layers: the parietal layer (lines the inside of the fibrous pericardium) and the visceral layer (adheres to the surface of the heart).

Between the fibrous and serous pericardium is the pericardial space. This space contains pericardial fluid, which lubricates the surfaces of the space and allows the heart to move easily during contraction.

Heart chambers

Within the heart lie four hollow chambers, two atria and two ventricles:

■ The right and left atria serve as volume reservoirs for blood being sent into the ventricles.

■ The interatrial septum divides the atrial chambers, helping them to contract and force blood into the ventricles below.

■ The ventricles serve as the pumping chambers of the heart.

■ The interventricular septum separates the ventricles and also helps them to pump.

Pump it up!

The thickness of a chamber's wall depends on the amount of high-pressure work the chamber does:

■ Because the atria only have to pump blood into the ventricles, their walls are relatively thin.

■ The walls of the **right ventricle** are thicker because it pumps blood against the resistance of the pulmonary circulation.

■ The walls of the **left ventricle** are thickest of all because it pumps blood against the resistance of the systemic circulation.

Inside a normal heart

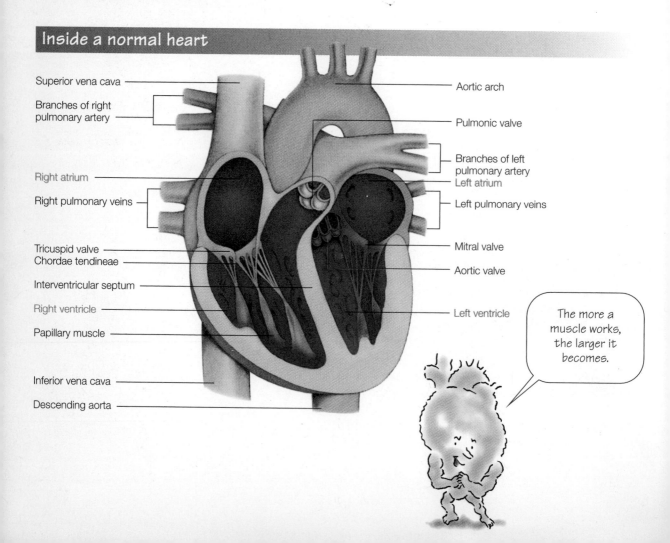

Superior vena cava

Branches of right pulmonary artery

Right atrium

Right pulmonary veins

Tricuspid valve
Chordae tendineae

Interventricular septum

Right ventricle

Papillary muscle

Inferior vena cava

Descending aorta

Aortic arch

Pulmonic valve

Branches of left pulmonary artery
Left atrium

Left pulmonary veins

Mitral valve

Aortic valve

Left ventricle

The more a muscle works, the larger it becomes.

Heart valves

The heart contains four valves: two atrioventricular (AV) valves (the mitral and tricuspid) and two semilunar valves (the pulmonic and aortic). The valves allow forward flow of blood through the heart and prevent backward flow.

The tricuspid valve, or right AV valve, prevents backflow from the right ventricle into the right atrium. The mitral valve, also known as the *bicuspid* or *left AV valve*, prevents backflow from the left ventricle into the left atrium. The pulmonic valve, one of the two semilunar valves, prevents backflow from the pulmonary artery into the right ventricle. The other semilunar valve is the aortic valve, which prevents backflow from the aorta into the left ventricle.

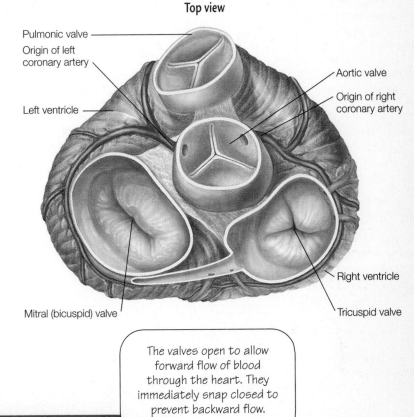

Top view

Pulmonic valve

Origin of left coronary artery

Left ventricle

Aortic valve

Origin of right coronary artery

Mitral (bicuspid) valve

Right ventricle

Tricuspid valve

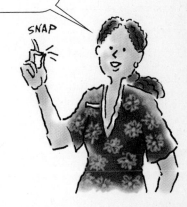

The valves open to allow forward flow of blood through the heart. They immediately snap closed to prevent backward flow.

SNAP

Under pressure!

Pressure changes within the heart affect the opening and closing of the valves. The amount of blood stretching the chamber and the degree of contraction of the chamber wall determine the pressure. For example, as blood fills a chamber, the pressure rises; then, as the chamber wall contracts, the pressure rises further. This increase in pressure causes the valve to open and blood to flow out into an area of lower pressure, leading to an equal pressure state.

Flow of blood through the heart

> Just like dancing a waltz, blood follows specific steps as it flows through the heart. One, two, three; one, two, three...

Step 1

Blood fills all heart chambers.
The right atrium receives deoxygenated blood returning from the body through the inferior and superior venae cavae and from the heart through the coronary sinus. The left atrium receives oxygenated blood from the lungs through the four pulmonary veins. Passive filling of the ventricles begins with diastole.

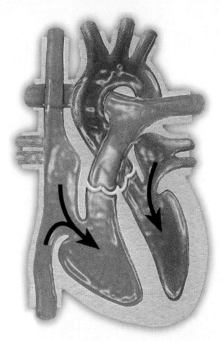

Step 2

The atria contract. The remaining blood enters the ventricles.
The atria pump their blood through the two AV valves (mitral and tricuspid) directly into their respective ventricles.

Step 3

The ventricles contract. Blood enters the aorta and pulmonary arteries.
The right ventricle pumps blood through the pulmonic valve into the pulmonary arteries and then into the lungs. That blood returns, oxygenated, to the left atrium, completing pulmonic circulation.

The left ventricle pumps blood through the aortic valve into the aorta and then throughout the body. Deoxygenated blood returns to the right atrium, completing systemic circulation.

Cardiac conduction

The conduction system of the heart begins with the heart's pacemaker: the sinoatrial (SA) node. When an impulse leaves the **SA node,** it travels through the atria along **Bachmann's bundle** and the **internodal pathways** on its way to the AV node. After the impulse passes through the **AV node,** it travels to the ventricles, first down the **bundle of His,** then along the **bundle branches** and, finally, down the **Purkinje fibers.**

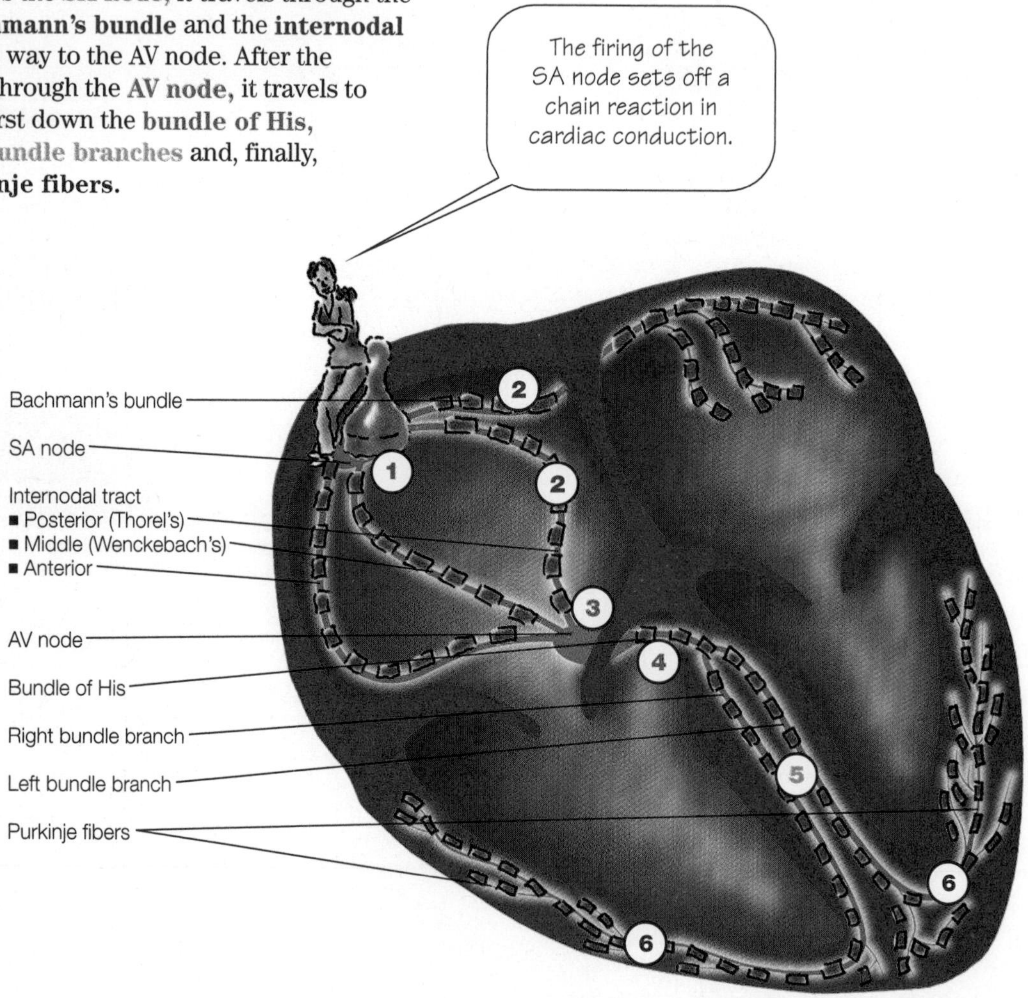

The firing of the SA node sets off a chain reaction in cardiac conduction.

Bachmann's bundle

SA node

Internodal tract
■ Posterior (Thorel's)
■ Middle (Wenckebach's)
■ Anterior

AV node

Bundle of His

Right bundle branch

Left bundle branch

Purkinje fibers

Pacemakers of the heart

The SA node is the heart's primary pacemaker. Pacemaker cells in lower areas, such as the junctional tissue and the Purkinje fibers, initiate an impulse only when they don't receive one from above, such as when the SA node is damaged from a myocardial infarction.

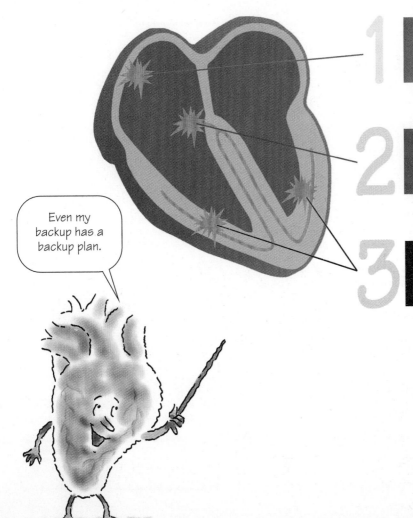

SA node
The SA node has a firing rate of 60 to 100 beats/minute.

AV node
The AV node has a firing rate of 40 to 60 beats/minute.

Purkinje fibers
The Purkinje fibers have a firing rate of 20 to 40 beats/minute.

Even my backup has a backup plan.

Generation and transmission of electrical impulses depend on four characteristics of cardiac cells.

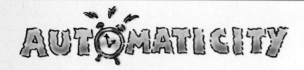

Ability to spontaneously initiate an impulse (pacemaker cells have this ability)

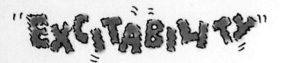

A cell's response to an electrical stimulus (results from ion shifts across the cell membrane)

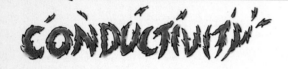

Ability of a cell to transmit an electrical impulse to another cardiac cell

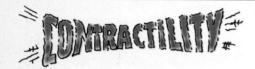

Ability of a cell to contract after receiving a stimulus

CONDUCTION JUNCTION

As impulses are transmitted, cardiac cells undergo cycles of depolarization and repolarization as described below.

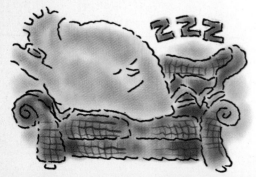

Our hero, the heart, is at rest, with no electrical activity taking place. He's enjoying the state of being polarized.

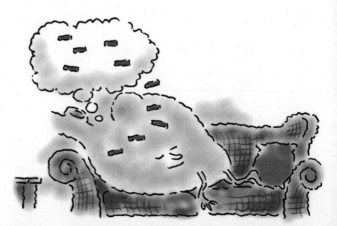

But while he rests, negative charges flow in, disturbing his rest. While he's still resting, he has the potential to react. This is his resting potential.

Depolarization-repolarization cycle

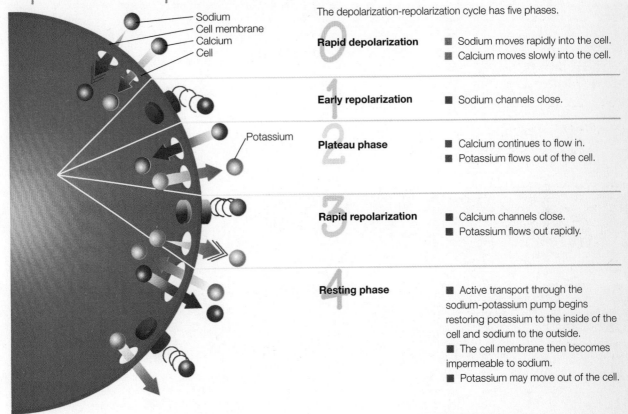

Sodium
Cell membrane
Calcium
Cell
Potassium

The depolarization-repolarization cycle has five phases.

0 Rapid depolarization
- Sodium moves rapidly into the cell.
- Calcium moves slowly into the cell.

1 Early repolarization
- Sodium channels close.

2 Plateau phase
- Calcium continues to flow in.
- Potassium flows out of the cell.

3 Rapid repolarization
- Calcium channels close.
- Potassium flows out rapidly.

4 Resting phase
- Active transport through the sodium-potassium pump begins restoring potassium to the inside of the cell and sodium to the outside.
- The cell membrane then becomes impermeable to sodium.
- Potassium may move out of the cell.

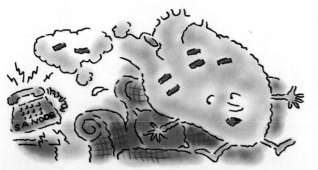

Disturbed by a ringing SA node, the ions of his dream state flow into his muscles. He has the potential for action and jumps from the sofa. This is his action potential. His cells have depolarized.

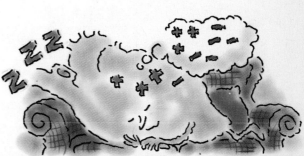

Wrong number. Our hero attempts to return to his resting state by balancing his negative experience with positive thoughts. He's trying to repolarize.

Cardiac output

Cardiac output refers to the amount of blood the heart pumps in 1 minute. To determine cardiac output, multiply the heart rate by the stroke volume (the amount of blood ejected with each heartbeat). Stroke volume depends on three factors:
- **preload**
- contractility
- afterload.

Preload is the stretching of muscle fibers in the ventricles as the ventricles fill with blood. Think of preload as a balloon stretching as air is blown into it. The more air being blown, the greater the stretch.

Contractility refers to the inherent ability of the myocardium to contract normally. Contractility is influenced by preload. The greater the stretch, the more forceful the contraction — or, the more air in the balloon, the greater the stretch, and the farther the balloon will fly when the air is allowed to expel.

Afterload refers to the pressure that the ventricular muscles must generate to overcome the higher pressure in the aorta to get the blood out of the heart. Resistance is the knot on the end of the balloon, which the balloon has to work against to get the air out.

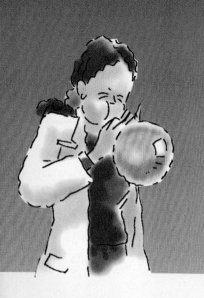

Wonder how the muscle contracts? Electrical stimulation causes troponin to expose actin-binding sites, which allows cardiac muscle contraction to occur.

Pulling it together

When a muscle cell is in the resting state, tropomyosin and troponin (a cardiac-specific protein) inhibit contractility by preventing actin-myosin binding.

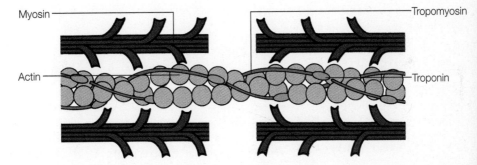

Myosin — Tropomyosin

Actin — Troponin

Electrical stimulation causes calcium release. Calcium binds to troponin, changing the configuration of tropomyosin and exposing actin-binding sites. Myosin and actin bind, creating cross-bridges, and the muscle contracts.

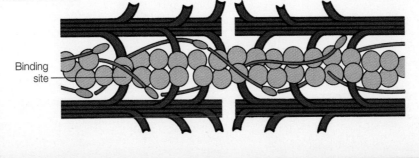

Binding site

Cycle of heart sounds

When you auscultate a patient's chest and hear that familiar "lub-dub," you're hearing the first and second heart sounds: S_1 and S_2. At times, two other sounds may occur: S_3 and S_4.

Heart sounds are generated by events in the cardiac cycle. When valves close or blood fills the ventricles, vibrations of the heart muscle can be heard through the chest wall.

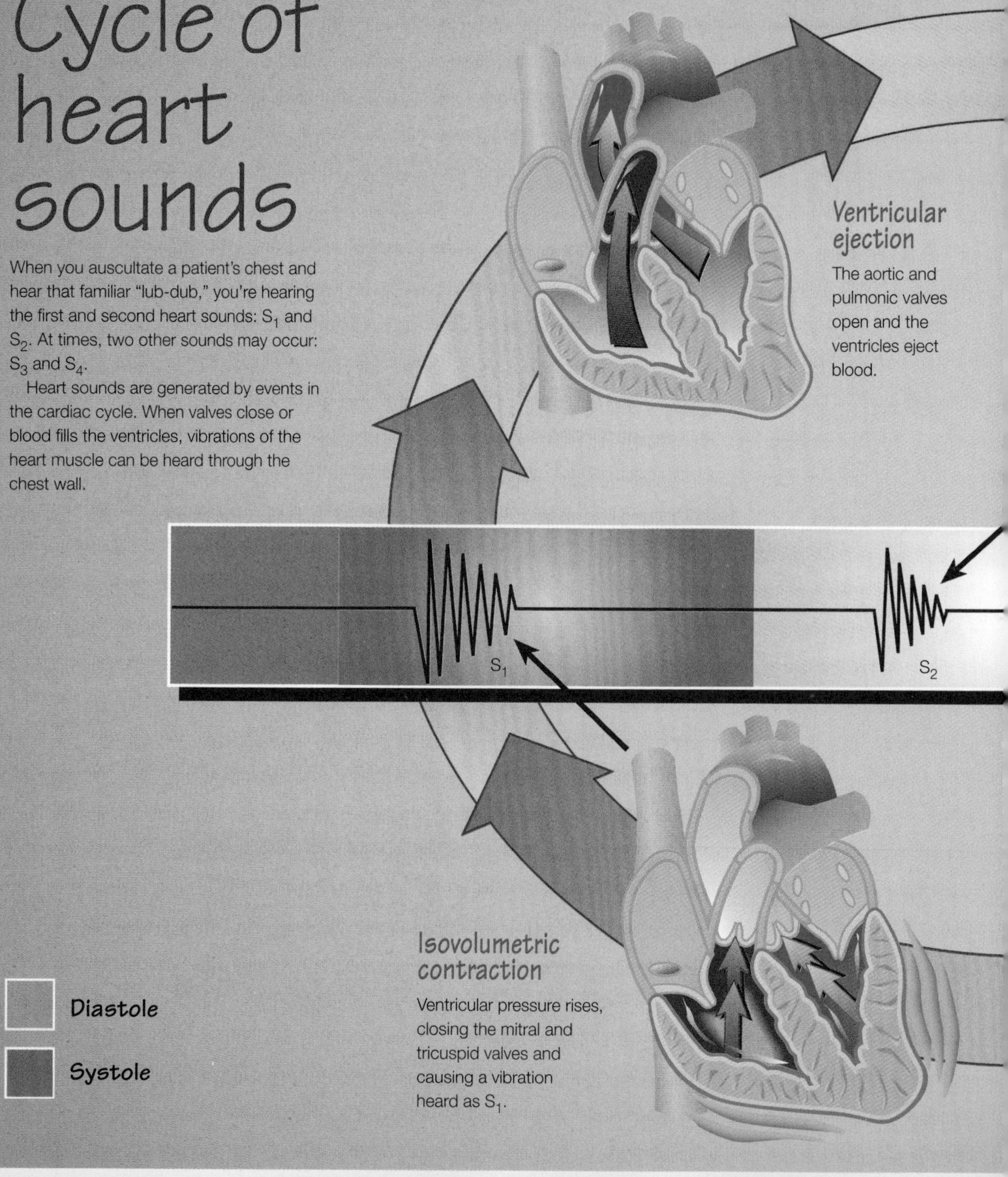

Ventricular ejection

The aortic and pulmonic valves open and the ventricles eject blood.

S_1

S_2

Isovolumetric contraction

Ventricular pressure rises, closing the mitral and tricuspid valves and causing a vibration heard as S_1.

☐ Diastole

■ Systole

Isometric relaxation

Ventricular pressure falls, and the aortic and pulmonic valves close, causing vibrations heard as S_2.

Rapid ventricular filling

Ventricular filling causes vibrations heard as S_3.

S_3 S_4

Slow ventricular filling

Atria contract and eject blood into resistant ventricles, causing vibrations heard as S_4.

Varying sound patterns

The phonogram at left shows how heart sounds vary in duration and intensity. For instance, S_2 (which occurs when the semilunar valves snap shut) is a shorter-lasting sound than S_1 because the semilunar valves take less time to close than the AV valves, which cause S_1.

Arteriovenous circulation

Blood flows through the body in five types of vessels:

■ *arteries* — have thick, muscular walls to accommodate high speed and pressure of blood flow

■ *arterioles* — have thinner walls than arteries; control blood flow to capillaries

■ *capillaries* — have microscopic walls composed of a single layer of endothelial cells

■ *venules* — gather blood from the capillaries; have thinner walls than arterioles

■ *veins* — have thinner walls but larger diameters than arteries.

Valves in the veins prevent blood backflow. Pressure from the moving volume of blood from below pushes pooled blood in each valved segment toward the heart.

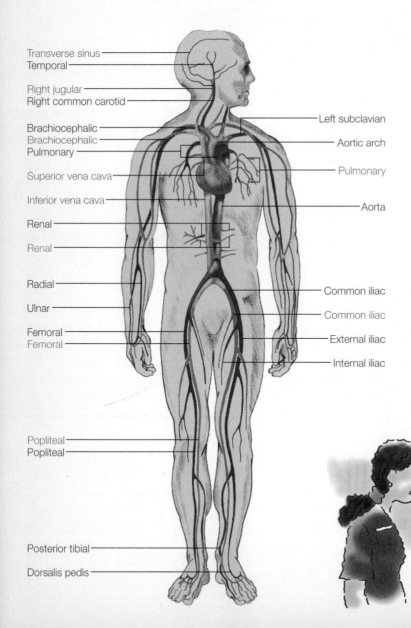

Transverse sinus
Temporal

Right jugular
Right common carotid

Brachiocephalic
Brachiocephalic
Pulmonary

Superior vena cava

Inferior vena cava

Renal

Renal

Radial

Ulnar

Femoral
Femoral

Popliteal
Popliteal

Posterior tibial

Dorsalis pedis

Left subclavian

Aortic arch

Pulmonary

Aorta

Common iliac

Common iliac

External iliac

Internal iliac

You think you're under pressure! Let me tell you what's going on in my world.

Blood circulation

Three methods of circulation carry blood throughout the body: pulmonary, systemic, and coronary.

4 ...and returns to the heart.

1 Blood leaves the heart...

3 ...exchanges nutrients and gases at the capillary level...

2 ...reaches a body structure...

Specialized circulatory systems

The circulatory system involves more than the circulation of blood out of the heart. The heart muscle itself—as well as the liver—must receive a steady supply of oxygenated blood.

Circulation to the heart muscle

The heart relies on the coronary arteries and their branches for its supply of oxygenated blood. It also depends on the cardiac veins to remove oxygen-depleted blood.

During diastole, blood flows out of the heart and into the coronary arteries. The right coronary artery supplies blood to the right atrium, part of the left atrium, most of the right ventricle, and the inferior part of the left ventricle. The left coronary artery, which splits into the anterior descending and circumflex arteries, supplies blood to the left atrium, most of the left ventricle, and most of the interventricular septum.

The cardiac veins lie superficial to the arteries. The largest vein, the coronary sinus, opens into the right atrium. Most of the major cardiac veins empty into the coronary sinus; the anterior cardiac veins, however, empty into the right atrium.

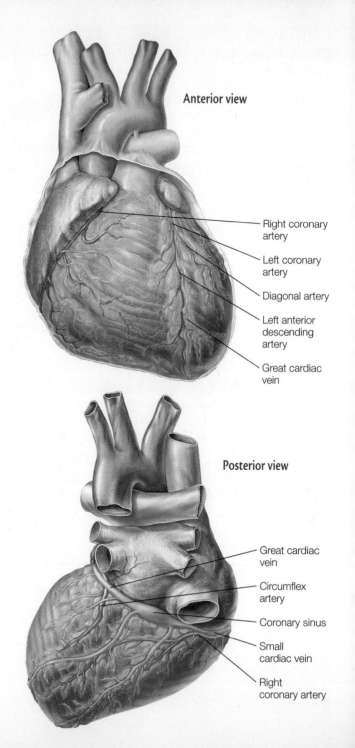

Anterior view

Right coronary artery

Left coronary artery

Diagonal artery

Left anterior descending artery

Great cardiac vein

Posterior view

Great cardiac vein

Circumflex artery

Coronary sinus

Small cardiac vein

Right coronary artery

Circulation to the liver

Seventy-five percent of the blood in the liver comes from the portal vein that drains the GI tract. This blood is full of nutrients. The other 25% is oxygenated blood that comes from the hepatic artery.

Capillary beds form the sinusoids of the liver, where hepatocytes filter and store nutrients and toxins. The sinusoids empty into the hepatic vein for venous return to the heart.

The circulation of blood into and out of the liver figures prominently in some disease processes.

Save the liver!

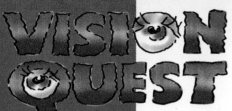

Able to label?

Label the heart chambers and heart valves indicated on this illustration.

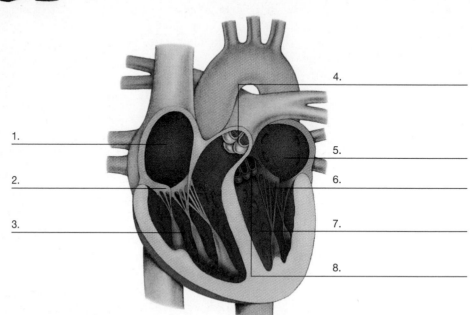

1. _____

2. _____

3. _____

4. _____

5. _____

6. _____

7. _____

8. _____

My word!

Unscramble the names of the five vessel types in the circulatory system. Then use the circled letters to answer the question posed.

Question: Which node is the heart's primary pacemaker?

1. elvesun _ _ O _ O _ _

2. areelsriot O _ O _ _ O _ _ _

3. siven _ _ O _ _

4. isacalliper _ O _ _ _ _ _ O _ _

5. eatersir _ O _ _ _ _ _ O

Answer: _ _ _ _ _ _ _ _ _ _

2 Assessment

Quiet on the set! The assessment is about to begin.

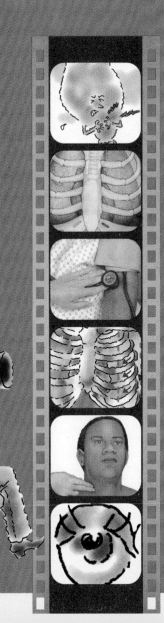

Taking a health history

The first step in assessing the cardiovascular system is to obtain a health history. Begin by introducing yourself and explaining what will occur during the health history and physical examination. Then ask about the patient's chief complaint. Also, be sure to ask about both the patient's personal and family health history.

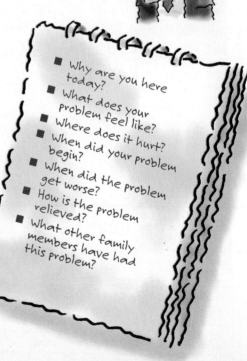

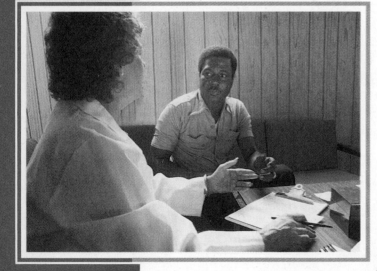

- Why are you here today?
- What does your problem feel like?
- Where does it hurt?
- When did your problem begin?
- When did the problem get worse?
- How is the problem relieved?
- What other family members have had this problem?

Common chief complaints

Chest pain

Many patients with cardiovascular problems complain at some point of chest pain. Chest pain can arise suddenly or gradually and can radiate to the arms, neck, jaw, or back. It can be steady or intermittent and mild or acute, and it can range in character from a sharp, shooting sensation to a feeling of heaviness, fullness, or even indigestion. The cause of chest pain may be difficult to determine at first. Chest pain can be provoked or aggravated by stress, anxiety, exertion, deep breathing, or consumption of certain foods.

> Steady or intermittent? Mild or acute? Sharp and shooting or heavy and full? Just trying to describe this chest pain is painful!

memory board

PQRST: What's the story?

Use the PQRST mnemonic to fully explore your patient's chest pain. When you ask the questions below, you'll encourage him to describe his symptom in greater detail. Remember to streamline your questions according to the patient's pain severity so that emergency care can be initiated promptly when indicated.

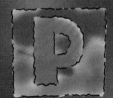 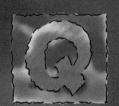 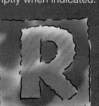 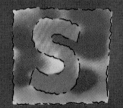 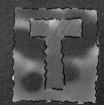

Provocative or palliative
- What provokes or relieves the chest pain?
- What makes the pain worsen or subside?

Quality or quantity
- What does the pain feel like?
- Are you having the pain right now? If so, is it more or less severe than usual?
- To what degree does chest pain affect your normal activities?

Region or radiation
- Where in the chest does the pain occur?
- Does the pain appear in other regions as well? If so, where?

Severity
- How severe is the chest pain? How would you rate it on a scale of 0 to 10, with 10 being the most severe?
- Does the pain seem to be diminishing, intensifying, or staying about the same?

Timing
- When did the pain begin?
- Was the onset sudden or gradual?
- How often does the pain occur?
- How long does it last?

Palpitations

Defined as a conscious awareness of one's heartbeat, palpitations are usually felt over the precordium or in the throat or neck. Palpitations may be regular or irregular, fast or slow, paroxysmal or sustained. Ask the patient to simulate his rhythm by tapping his finger on a hard surface.

      Most palpitations are insignificant. However, they can be caused by such disorders as arrhythmias, hypertension, mitral prolapse, and mitral stenosis.

> Are you sure that's what your palpitations feel like? That sounds an awful lot like "Jingle Bells."

Ask the patient the following questions about his palpitations:
- What are your palpitations like? For example, are they pounding, jumping, fluttering, or flopping?
- Do you have a sensation of missed or skipped beats?
- Do you have a history of hypertension?
- Have you recently started digoxin therapy?
- What medications do you take?
- Do you smoke, drink caffeinated beverages, or consume alcohol? If so, how much?

Syncope

Syncope is a brief loss of consciousness caused by a lack of blood to the brain. It usually occurs abruptly and can last for seconds to minutes. It may result from such disorders as aortic arch syndrome, aortic stenosis, and arrhythmias.

      When syncope occurs, the patient typically lies motionless, with his skeletal muscles relaxed. The depth of unconsciousness varies. The patient is strikingly pale with a slow, weak pulse; hypotension; and almost imperceptible breathing.

Ask the patient the following questions about his syncope:
- Did you feel weak, lightheaded, nauseous, or sweaty just before you fainted?
- Did you get up quickly from a chair or from lying down?
- During the fainting episode, did you have muscle spasms or incontinence?
- How long were you unconscious?
- When you regained consciousness, were you alert or confused?
- Did you have a headache?
- Have you fainted before? If so, how often do the episodes occur?

> Hmm...He's pale and motionless; has a slow, weak pulse and hypotension; and is barely breathing. I'd say he isn't getting enough blood to his brain.

Intermittent claudication really cramps my lifestyle.

Intermittent claudication

Intermittent claudication is cramping limb pain that's brought on by exercise and relieved by 1 or 2 minutes of rest. It usually occurs in the legs. This pain may be acute or chronic; when acute, it may signal acute arterial occlusion. Intermittent claudication typically results from such disorders as aortic arteriosclerotic occlusive disease, acute arterial occlusion, or arteriosclerosis obliterans.

Ask the patient the following questions about his intermittent claudication:
- How far can you walk before pain occurs?
- How long must you rest before it subsides?
- Can you walk as far as you could before, or must you rest more often?
- Does the pain-rest pattern vary?
- Has this symptom affected your lifestyle?

Peripheral edema

Peripheral edema results from excess interstitial fluid in the arms or legs. It may be unilateral or bilateral, slight or dramatic, and pitting or nonpitting. Arm edema may be caused by superior vena cava syndrome or thrombophlebitis. Leg edema may be an early sign of right-sided heart failure, thrombophlebitis, or chronic venous insufficiency.

Ask the patient the following questions about his peripheral edema:
- How long have you had the edema?
- Did it develop suddenly or gradually?
- Does the edema decrease if you elevate your extremity?
- Is it worse in the mornings, or does it progressively worsen during the day?
- Did you recently injure the affected extremity or have surgery or an illness that caused you to be immobile?
- Do you have a history of cardiovascular disease?
- Are you taking prescription or over-the-counter medications?

Other signs and symptoms

Next, inquire about the patient's family history and past medical history, including history of heart disease, diabetes, or chronic lung, kidney, or liver disease.

Ask the patient with cardiovascular complaints if he has any of these signs or symptoms:
- shortness of breath on exertion, when lying down, or at night
- cough
- cyanosis or pallor
- weakness
- fatigue
- unexplained weight change
- dizziness
- headache
- high or low blood pressure
- peripheral skin changes, such as decreased hair distribution, skin color changes, or a thin, shiny appearance to the skin.

I know it seems like we've been here a long time, but I'm almost done.

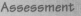

Measuring blood pressure

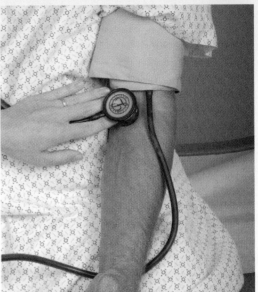

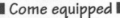

Come equipped

When you take a patient's blood pressure, you're measuring the lateral force that blood exerts on the arterial walls as the heart contracts (systolic pressure) and relaxes (diastolic pressure). Use these tips to obtain the most accurate reading:

- Use a cuff that's 20% to 25% wider than the patient's arm circumference.
- Support the patient's arm at heart level.
- Use the bell of the stethoscope.
- Deflate the cuff at 2 to 3 mm Hg per second.
- Listen for the five phases of Korotkoff sounds.

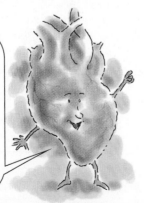

Record the systolic blood pressure when you hear the first two consecutive sounds of phase I. With the onset of silence in phase V, record the diastolic pressure.

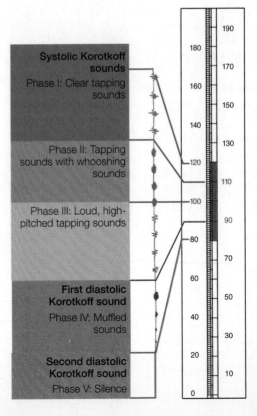

Systolic Korotkoff sounds

Phase I: Clear tapping sounds

Phase II: Tapping sounds with whooshing sounds

Phase III: Loud, high-pitched tapping sounds

First diastolic Korotkoff sound

Phase IV: Muffled sounds

Second diastolic Korotkoff sound

Phase V: Silence

Performing cardiac inspection

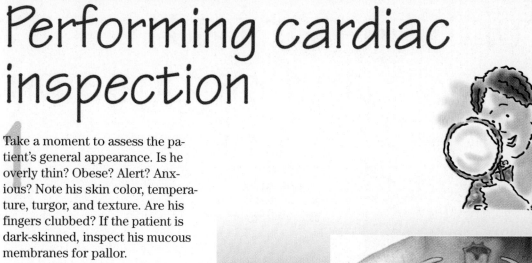

Take a moment to assess the patient's general appearance. Is he overly thin? Obese? Alert? Anxious? Note his skin color, temperature, turgor, and texture. Are his fingers clubbed? If the patient is dark-skinned, inspect his mucous membranes for pallor.

Next, inspect the chest. Note landmarks you can use to describe your findings and to identify structures underlying the chest wall. Also look for pulsations, symmetry of movement, retractions, or heaves (a strong outward thrust of the chest wall that occurs during systole).

Note the location of the apical impulse. You should find it in the fifth intercostal space, medial to the left midclavicular line. Because it corresponds to the apex of the heart, the apical pulse helps indicate how well the left ventricle is working. The apical pulse is usually the point of maximal impulse. It can be seen in about 50% of adults. You'll notice it more easily in children and in patients with thin chest walls.

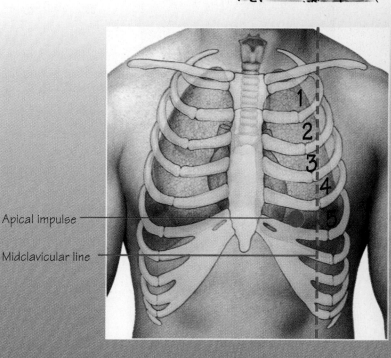

Apical impulse

Midclavicular line

Performing cardiac palpation and percussion

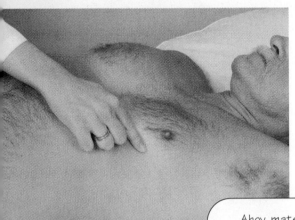

Maintain a gentle touch when you palpate so that you don't obscure pulsations or similar findings. Using the ball of your hand, then your fingertips, palpate over the precordium to find the apical impulse. Note heaves or thrills (fine vibrations that feel like the purring of a cat).

The apical impulse may be difficult to palpate in an obese or a pregnant patient and in a patient with a thick chest wall. If it's difficult to palpate with the patient lying on his back, have him lie on his left side or sit upright. It may also be helpful to have the patient exhale completely and hold his breath for a few seconds.

Ahoy, matey. Follow the percussion map to help you find your way on your assessment journey. Listen closely, though, to make sure you're on the right path.

Anterior axillary line

Heart border

Fifth intercostal space

Start here

Midclavicular line

Begin percussing at the anterior axillary line, moving toward the sternum along the third, fourth, and fifth intercostal spaces. The sound changes from resonance to dullness over the left border of the heart, normally at the midclavicular line. The right border of the heart is usually aligned with the sternum and can't be percussed.

Auscultating for heart sounds

Cardiac auscultation requires a methodical approach and lots of practice. Begin by identifying the four auscultation sites. Auscultation sites are identified by the names of heart valves but aren't located directly over the valves. Rather, these sites are located along the pathway blood takes as it flows through the heart's chambers and valves.

> You can learn a great deal about the heart by auscultating for heart sounds.

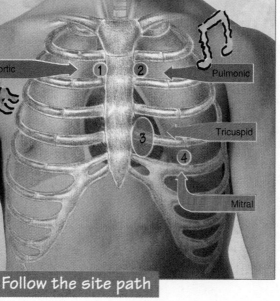

Aortic   1   2   Pulmonic

3   Tricuspid

4

Mitral

1 Begin auscultating over the **aortic area,** placing the stethoscope over the second intercostal space, along the right sternal border.

2 Then move to the **pulmonic area,** located at the second intercostal space, at the left sternal border.

3 Next, assess the **tricuspid area,** which lies over the fourth and fifth intercostal spaces, along the left sternal border.

4 Finally, listen over the **mitral area,** located at the fifth intercostal space, near the midclavicular line.

Follow the site path

■ In the **aortic area,** sounds reflect blood moving from the left ventricle during systole, crossing the aortic valve, and flowing through the aortic arch.
■ In the **pulmonic area,** sounds reflect blood being ejected from the right ventricle during systole and then crossing the pulmonic valve and flowing through the main pulmonary artery.
■ In the **tricuspid area,** sounds reflect movement of blood from the right atrium across the tricuspid valve and right ventricular filling during diastole.
■ In the **mitral area,** also called the *apical area,* sounds reflect blood flow across the mitral valve and left ventricular filling during diastole.

Heart sounds

Systole is the period of ventricular contraction. As pressure in the ventricles increases, the mitral and tricuspid valves snap closed. That closure produces the first heart sound, S_1. At the end of ventricular contraction, the aortic and pulmonic valves snap shut. This produces the second heart sound, S_2.

Always identify S_1 and S_2, and then listen for adventitious sounds, such as third and fourth heart sounds (S_3 and S_4). Also listen for murmurs, which sound like vibrating, blowing, or rumbling noises.

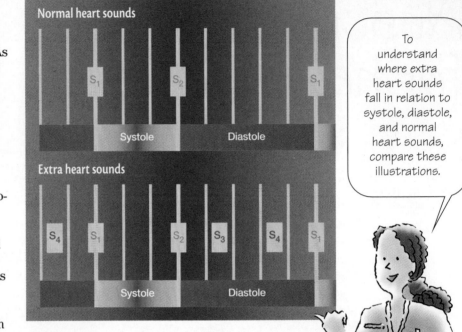

Normal heart sounds

S_1 S_2 S_1

Systole   Diastole

Extra heart sounds

S_4 S_1 S_2 S_3 S_4 S_1

Systole   Diastole

To understand where extra heart sounds fall in relation to systole, diastole, and normal heart sounds, compare these illustrations.

Auscultation tips

■ Concentrate as you listen for each sound.
■ Avoid auscultating through clothing or wound dressings because these items can block sound.
■ Avoid picking up extraneous sounds by keeping the stethoscope tubing off the patient's body and other surfaces.
■ Until you become proficient at auscultation, explain to the patient that listening to his chest for a long period doesn't mean that anything is wrong.
■ Ask the patient to breathe normally and to hold his breath periodically to enhance sounds that may be difficult to hear.

Identifying abnormal heart sounds

Murmurs

Murmurs can occur during systole or diastole and are described by several criteria. Their pitch can be high, medium, or low. They can vary in intensity or configuration, growing louder or softer. They can vary by location, sound pattern (blowing, harsh, or musical), radiation (to the neck or axillae), and period during which they occur in the cardiac cycle (pansystolic, midsystolic, or diastolic).

More on murmurs

If you identify a heart murmur, listen closely to determine its timing in the cardiac cycle. Then determine its other characteristics: quality (blowing, musical, harsh, or rumbling), pitch (medium, high, or low), and location (where the murmur sounds the loudest). Use a standard, six-level grading scale to describe the intensity (loudness) of the murmur.

Grade 1—barely audible, even to the trained ear

Grade 2—clearly audible

Grade 3—moderately loud

Grade 4—loud with palpable thrill

Grade 5—very loud with a palpable thrill; can be heard when the stethoscope has only partial contact with the chest

Grade 6—extremely loud with a palpable thrill; can be heard with the stethoscope lifted just off the chest wall

photo op

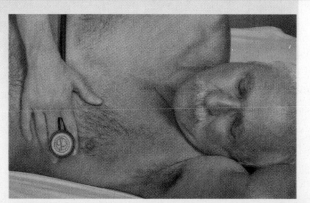

The best way to hear murmurs is with the patient sitting up and leaning forward or lying on his left side, as shown at left. Listen for murmurs over the same precordial areas used in auscultation for heart sounds.

Murmur configurations

To help classify a murmur, begin by identifying its configuration (shape). Shown below are four basic patterns of murmurs.

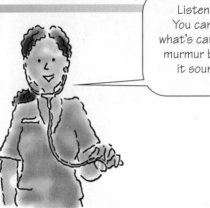

Listen up! You can tell what's causing a murmur by how it sounds.

Crescendo/decrescendo
(diamond-shaped)
- Begins softly, peaks sharply, and then fades
- Examples: Pulmonic stenosis, aortic stenosis, mitral valve prolapse, mitral stenosis

Decrescendo
- Starts loudly and then gradually diminishes
- Examples: Aortic insufficiency, pulmonic insufficiency

Pansystolic
(holosystolic or plateau-shaped)
- Is uniform from beginning to end
- Examples: Mitral or tricuspid regurgitation

Crescendo
- Begins softly and then gradually increases
- Examples: Tricuspid stenosis, mitral valve prolapse

Differentiating murmurs

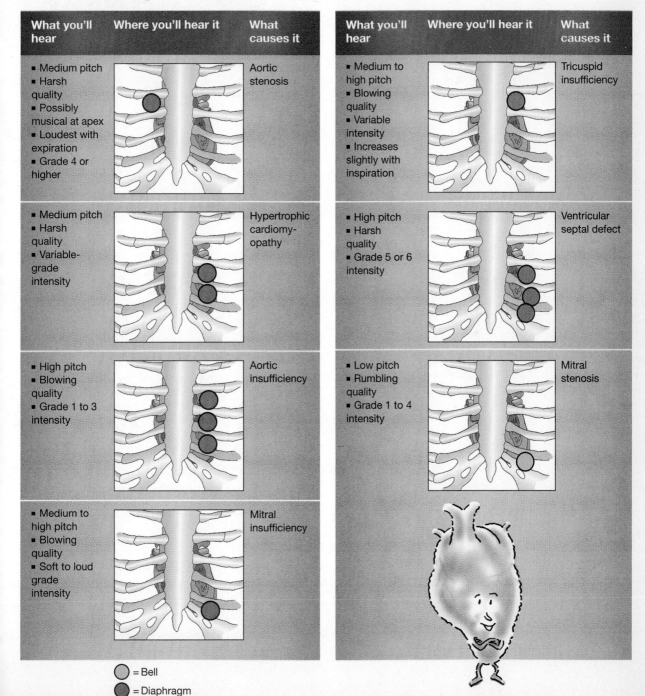

What you'll hear	Where you'll hear it	What causes it
• Medium pitch • Harsh quality • Possibly musical at apex • Loudest with expiration • Grade 4 or higher		Aortic stenosis
• Medium pitch • Harsh quality • Variable-grade intensity		Hypertrophic cardiomy-opathy
• High pitch • Blowing quality • Grade 1 to 3 intensity		Aortic insufficiency
• Medium to high pitch • Blowing quality • Soft to loud grade intensity		Mitral insufficiency

What you'll hear	Where you'll hear it	What causes it
• Medium to high pitch • Blowing quality • Variable intensity • Increases slightly with inspiration		Tricuspid insufficiency
• High pitch • Harsh quality • Grade 5 or 6 intensity		Ventricular septal defect
• Low pitch • Rumbling quality • Grade 1 to 4 intensity		Mitral stenosis

⬤ = Bell

⬤ = Diaphragm

Gallops and rubs

S₃: Classic sign of heart failure

S₃, also known as *ventricular gallop*, is commonly heard in children and may be normal in patients during the last trimester of pregnancy; however, it may be a cardinal sign of heart failure in other adults. Because it follows S₂, it's commonly compared to the "y" sound in "Ken-tuck-y." S₃ is low-pitched; you'll hear it best at the apex when the patient is lying on his left side.

■ In early ventricular diastole, the pulmonic and aortic valves snap closed, producing S₂.

■ A large amount of blood rushes into the ventricles, possibly as a result of pulmonary edema, an atrial septal defect, or an acute myocardial infarction (MI).

■ The rapid ventricular filling causes vibrations, producing S₃.

S₄: An MI aftereffect

Also called an *atrial gallop*, S₄ is an adventitious heart sound that you'll hear best over the tricuspid or mitral area when the patient lies on his left side. Patients who are elderly and those with hypertension, aortic stenosis, or a history of MI may have an S₄. It's commonly described as sounding like "Ten-nes-see" because it occurs just before S₁, after atrial contraction.

■ In atrial diastole, the atria contract to eject blood into the ventricles.

■ If the ventricles don't move or expand as much as they should, the atria must work harder to eject the blood. This causes the atria to vibrate, producing a sound known as S₄.

■ As the ventricles fill and pressure rises, the mitral and tricuspid valves snap close, producing S₁.

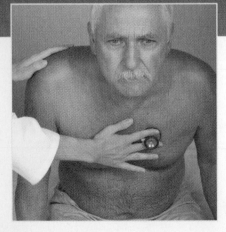

Don't rub me the wrong way!

Listening for pericardial friction rub is also an important part of your assessment. To do this, have the patient sit upright, lean forward, and exhale, as shown at left. Listen with the diaphragm of the stethoscope over the third intercostal space on the left side of the chest. A pericardial friction rub has a scratchy, rubbing quality. If you suspect a rub but have trouble hearing one, ask the patient to hold his breath.

Assessing the vascular system

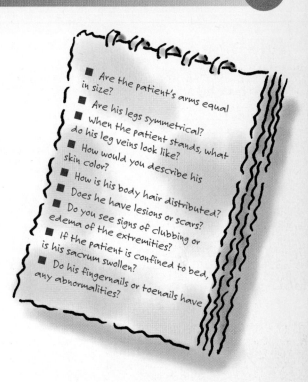

Inspection

Start your assessment of the vascular system the same way you start an assessment of the cardiac system — by making general observations. For example, begin by examining the patient's arms when you take his vital signs. Complete your inspection by using the checklist at right.

- Are the patient's arms equal in size?
- Are his legs symmetrical?
- When the patient stands, what do his leg veins look like?
- How would you describe his skin color?
- How is his body hair distributed?
- Does he have lesions or scars?
- Do you see signs of clubbing or edema of the extremities?
- If the patient is confined to bed, is his sacrum swollen?
- Do his fingernails or toenails have any abnormalities?

Assessing jugular vein distention

Now inspect the jugular veins. The internal jugular vein has a softer, undulating pulsation. Unlike the pulsation of the carotid artery, pulsation of the internal jugular vein changes in response to position, breathing, and palpation. The vein normally protrudes when the patient is lying down and lies flat when he stands.

When jugular vein distention is detected, measure it with a horizontal straight edge aligned with the top of the pulsations. Then read the vertical distance on a ruler. A measurement of 3 to 4 cm above the sternal angle is abnormal.

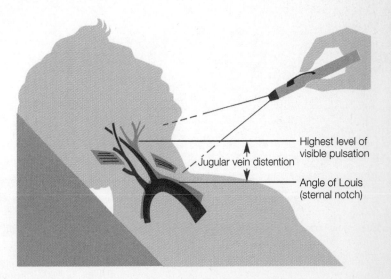

Highest level of visible pulsation

Jugular vein distention

Angle of Louis (sternal notch)

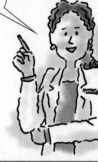

To assess arterial pulses, apply pressure with your index and middle fingers.

Palpation

The next step in an assessment of the vascular system is to palpate the arterial pulses. All pulses should be regular in rhythm and equal in strength.

Carotid pulse

Lightly place your fingers just medial to the trachea and below the jaw angle. Never palpate both carotid arteries at the same time.

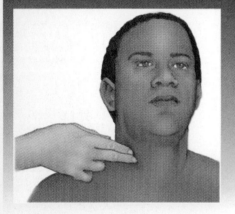

Brachial pulse

Position your fingers medial to the biceps tendon.

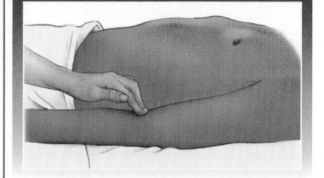

Making the grade

Pulses are graded on the following scale:

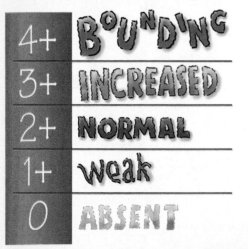

4+ BOUNDING
3+ INCREASED
2+ NORMAL
1+ weak
0 ABSENT

Radial pulse

Apply gentle pressure to the medial and ventral side of the wrist, just below the base of the thumb.

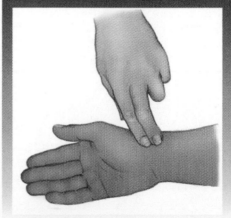

A 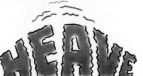 **HEAVE**, lifting of the chest wall felt during palpation along the left sternal border, may mean right ventricular hypertrophy; over the left ventricular area, a ventricular aneurysm.

A **THRILL**, which is a palpable vibration, usually suggests valvular dysfunction.

Dorsalis pedis pulse

Place your fingers on the medial dorsum of the foot while the patient points his toes down. The pulse is difficult to palpate here and may appear absent in a healthy patient.

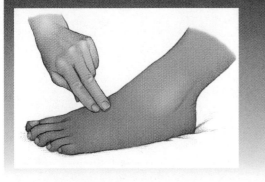

Femoral pulse

Press relatively hard at a point inferior to the inguinal ligament. For an obese patient, palpate in the crease of the groin, halfway between the pubic bone and the hip bone.

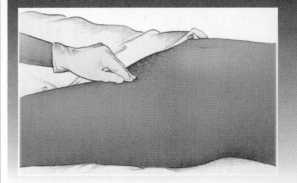

Posterior tibial pulse

Apply pressure behind and slightly below the malleolus of the ankle.

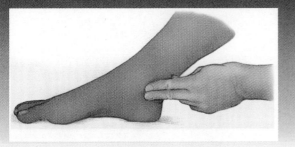

Popliteal pulse

Press firmly in the popliteal fossa at the back of the knee.

Auscultation

Following the palpation sequence and using the bell of the stethoscope, listen over each artery. You shouldn't hear sounds over the carotid arteries. A bruit sounds like buzzing or blowing and could indicate arteriosclerotic plaque formation.

   Assess the upper abdomen for abnormal pulsations, which could indicate the presence of an abdominal aortic aneurysm. Finally, auscultate the renal, iliac, femoral, and aortic pulses, checking for a bruit or other abnormal sounds.

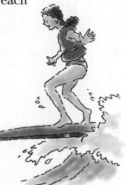

Let's catch some waves!

To identify abnormal arterial pulses, check the waveforms below and see which one matches your patient's peripheral pulse.

Weak pulse

A weak pulse has a decreased amplitude with a slower upstroke and downstroke. Possible causes of a weak pulse include increased peripheral vascular resistance, as occurs in cold weather or with severe heart failure, and decreased stroke volume, as occurs with hypovolemia or aortic stenosis.

Bounding pulse

A bounding pulse has a sharp upstroke and downstroke with a pointed peak and elevated amplitude. Possible causes of bounding pulse include increased stroke volume, as with aortic insufficiency, or arterial wall stiffness, which can occur with aging.

Pulsus alternans

Pulsus alternans has a regular, alternating pattern of weak and strong pulses. This pulse is associated with left-sided heart failure.

Pulsus bigeminus

Pulsus bigeminus is similar to pulsus alternans but occurs at irregular intervals. This pulse is caused by premature atrial or ventricular beats.

Pulsus paradoxus

Pulsus paradoxus has increases and decreases in amplitude associated with the respiratory cycle. Marked decreases occur when the patient inhales. Pulsus paradoxus is associated with pericardial tamponade, advanced heart failure, and constrictive pericarditis.

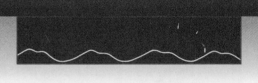

Inspiration   Expiration

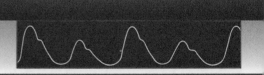

Pulsus biferiens

Pulsus biferiens shows an initial upstroke, a subsequent downstroke, and then another upstroke during systole. Pulsus biferiens is caused by aortic stenosis and aortic insufficiency.

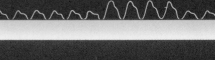

Abdominal auscultation points

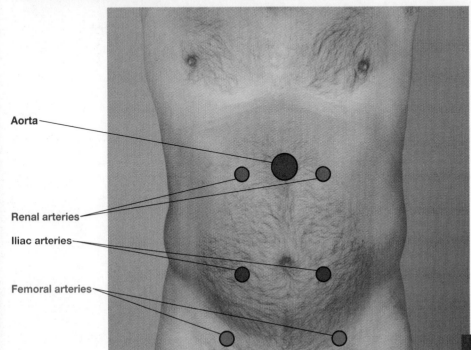

Aorta

Renal arteries

Iliac arteries

Femoral arteries

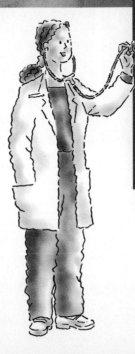

What's all the bruit ha ha?

If the patient has hypertension, you may hear a bruit—a vascular sound similar to a heart murmur that is caused by turbulent blood flow through a narrowed artery. Occasionally, you may hear a bruit limited to systole in the epigastric region of a healthy person.

Identifying abnormal vascular findings

Peripheral edema

Edema (swelling) may indicate heart failure or venous insufficiency. It may also be caused by varicosities or thrombophlebitis.

Pitting edema is swelling, usually of venous origin, that results in a pit or depression in the affected area when a thumb is pressed firmly but gently into the skin for at least 5 seconds. Swelling caused primarily by lymph fluid collection in a dependent area may not cause pitting.

If a patient has nonpitting edema in an extremity, measure the circumference of the affected and unaffected limbs and compare the difference. Take measurements regularly to detect changes.

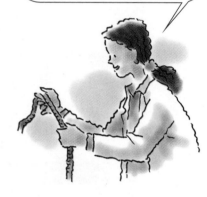

It's the pits!

Pitting edema is graded on a 4-point scale.

0 = no pitting although edema may be present

+1 = 2 mm indentation

+2 = 4 mm indentation

+3 = 6 mm indentation

+4 = 8 mm indentation

Vascular insufficiency

Assessment findings differ in patients with arterial insufficiency and those with chronic venous insufficiency.

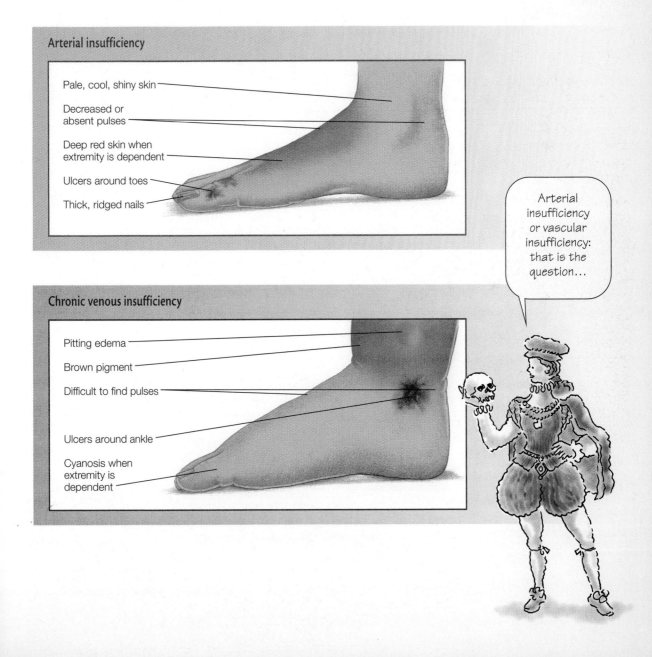

Arterial insufficiency

Pale, cool, shiny skin

Decreased or absent pulses

Deep red skin when extremity is dependent

Ulcers around toes

Thick, ridged nails

Chronic venous insufficiency

Pitting edema

Brown pigment

Difficult to find pulses

Ulcers around ankle

Cyanosis when extremity is dependent

Arterial insufficiency or vascular insufficiency: that is the question...

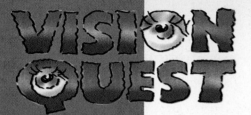

Matchmaker

Match the murmur configuration shown with the name that describes it.

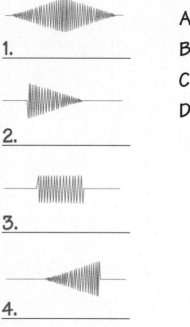

1. _____

2. _____

3. _____

4. _____

A. Decrescendo

B. Crescendo

C. Pansystolic

D. Crescendo/decrescendo

Able to label?

Identify the signs and symptoms of arterial insufficiency indicated on this illustration.

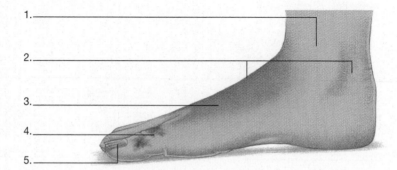

1. _____

2. _____

3. _____

4. _____

5. _____

3 Diagnostic tests

The results of diagnostic tests help to direct your patient's care.

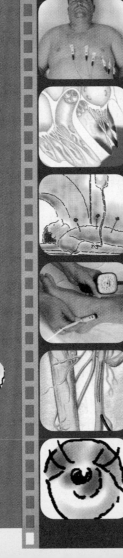

Blood tests

Tests to identify myocardial infarction

After a myocardial infarction (MI), damaged cardiac tissue releases significant amounts of enzymes and proteins into the blood. Specific blood tests help reveal the extent of cardiac damage and help monitor healing progress.

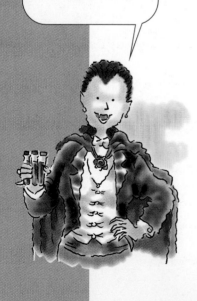

I vant to test your blood! Some blood tests, such as cardiac enzyme and protein tests, evaluate damage to the heart muscle. Other tests help to identify patients at risk for heart disease.

- **Myoglobin**
  - Elevated
  - First marker of cardiac injury after acute MI
- **CK-MB**
  - Returns to normal quickly
  - Most reliable when reported as a percentage of total CK (relative index)
- **LD_1 and LD_2**
  - Isoenzymes of lactate dehydrogenase (LD)
  - Flipped LD levels ($LD_1 > LD_2$)
  - Less frequently used as test
- **Troponin I**
  - Isotype of troponin found only in myocardium
  - Elevated
  - Specific to myocardial damage
- **Troponin T**
  - Isotype of troponin that's less specific to myocardial damage (can indicate renal failure)
  - Elevated
  - Determined quickly at bedside

Values

Myoglobin
- Normal value: 0 to 0.09 mcg/ml
- Rises within 30 minutes to 4 hours
- Peaks within 6 to 10 hours
- Returns to baseline by 24 hours

CK-MB
- Normal value: 38 to 190 units/L for men; 10 to 150 units/L for women
- Rises within 4 to 8 hours
- Peaks in 12 to 24 hours
- May remain elevated for up to 96 hours

LD$_1$-LD$_2$
- Normal value: 35 to 378 units/L (depending on the methods used)
- Rises within 12 to 24 hours
- Peaks in 2 to 5 days
- Returns to normal in 7 to 14 days (if tissue necrosis doesn't persist)

Troponin I
- Normal value: Less than 0.4 mcg/ml (may vary depending on the laboratory)
- Rises within 4 to 6 hours
- Peaks in 10 to 24 hours
- Returns to baseline in 3 to 10 days

Troponin T
- Normal value: Less than 0.1 mcg/ml (may vary depending on the laboratory)
- Rises within 4 to 6 hours
- Peaks in 12 to 48 hours
- Returns to baseline in 7 to 10 days

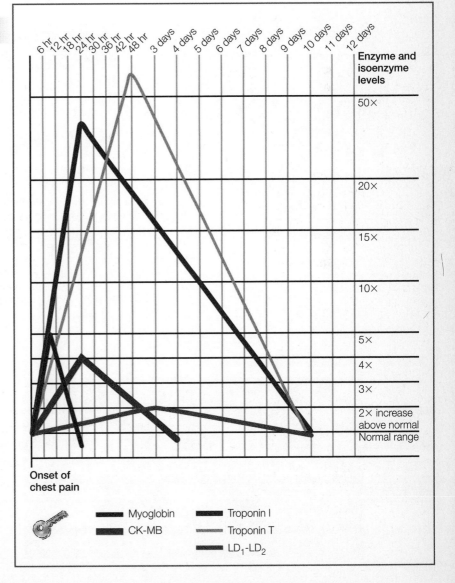

Onset of chest pain

Enzyme and isoenzyme levels: 50×, 20×, 15×, 10×, 5×, 4×, 3×, 2× increase above normal, Normal range

Time axis: 6 hr, 12 hr, 18 hr, 24 hr, 30 hr, 36 hr, 42 hr, 48 hr, 3 days, 4 days, 5 days, 6 days, 7 days, 8 days, 9 days, 10 days, 11 days, 12 days

Key:
- Myoglobin
- CK-MB
- Troponin I
- Troponin T
- LD$_1$-LD$_2$

Tests to identify the risk of heart disease

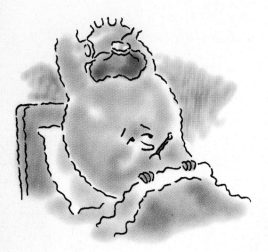

Homocysteine (tHcy)

- Normal value: ≤ 13 μmol/L
- Excess levels
  - Irritate blood vessels, leading to atherosclerosis
  - Raise low-density lipoprotein (LDL) levels
  - Make blood clot more easily

High-sensitivity C-reactive protein (hs-CRP)

- Normal value: 0.02 to 0.8 mg/dl
- Excess levels: May indicate increased risk of coronary artery disease (CAD)

Triglycerides

- Normal value: < 150 mg/dl
- Excess levels: Help with early identification of hyperlipidemia and identification of patients at risk for CAD

Total cholesterol

- Normal value: < 200 mg/dl for adults; < 170 mg/dl for children and adolescents
- Excess levels: May indicate hereditary lipid disorders, CAD

Evaluating lipid test results

Use this chart to determine an adult patient's risk of CAD.

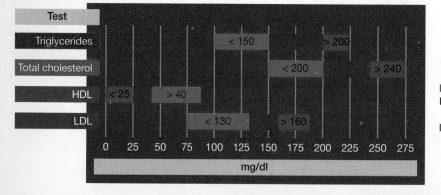

Test											
Triglycerides				< 150		> 200					
Total cholesterol					< 200		> 240				
HDL	< 25	> 40									
LDL			< 130		> 160						

0 25 50 75 100 125 150 175 200 225 250 275

mg/dl

- Desirable level — No treatment
- Borderline level — May need conservative treatment
- High risk of CAD — Requires careful medical management

Lipoprotein fractionation

Lipoprotein fractionation tests isolate and measure high-density lipoproteins (HDLs), LDLs, and very-low-density lipoproteins (VLDLs). Each of these particles is composed of protein, cholesterol, and triglyceride in varying amounts.

HDL

- Primarily protein
- Test measures the actual amount in the blood
- The *higher* the level, the *lower* the risk of CAD
- Normal values for males: 37 to 70 mg/dl; for females, 40 to 85 mg/dl

LDL

- Mainly cholesterol
- Equal to total cholesterol – HDL cholesterol – VLDL cholesterol (when triglyceride level is below 400 mg/dl)
- The *higher* the LDL level, the *higher* the incidence of CAD
- Normal levels for individuals without CAD, < 130 mg/dl
- Optimal levels for individuals with CAD, < 100 mg/dl

VLDL

- Mainly triglycerides
- Calculated as triglyceride level ÷ 5
- The *higher* the VLDL level, the *higher* the incidence of CAD
- Can be measured with a more sensitive test when high-risk patients and those with triglyceride levels of 400 mg/dl or more require complex medical management

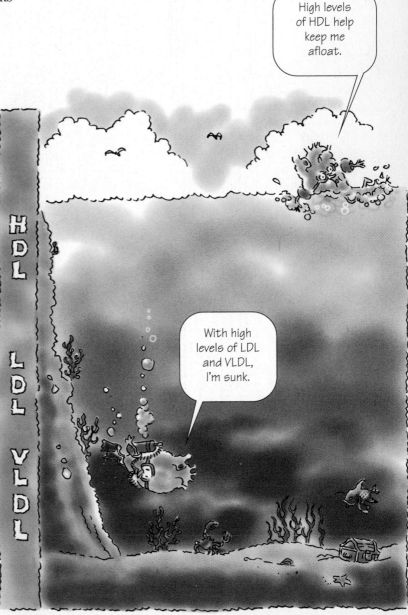

Tests to identify the risk of heart failure

Heart cells produce and store two neurohormones — A-type natriuretic peptide (ANP) and B-type natriuretic peptide (BNP) — that help ensure cardiac equilibrium. Disruptions in fluid balance within the circulatory system trigger release of these hormones, which act as natural diuretics and antihypertensives.

ANP

- Found in atrial tissue
- Nornal value: 20 to 77 pg/ml

BNP

- Found in ventricular tissue
- Helps accurately diagnose and grade heart failure severity
- Normal value: < 100 pg/ml

ANP is released by the atria in response to acute increased fluid volume and pressure.

The atria and ventricles become enlarged in response to increased fluid volume.

BNP is released by the ventricles in response to prolonged fluid volume overload or elevated pressure.

Correlating the degree of heart failure with BNP level

The higher a patient's level of BNP, the greater the degree of heart failure. In turn, the greater the degree of heart failure, the more the patient's ability to perform activities of daily living (ADLs) will be impaired. Use this chart to help you plan your nursing care.

New York Heart Association Classification

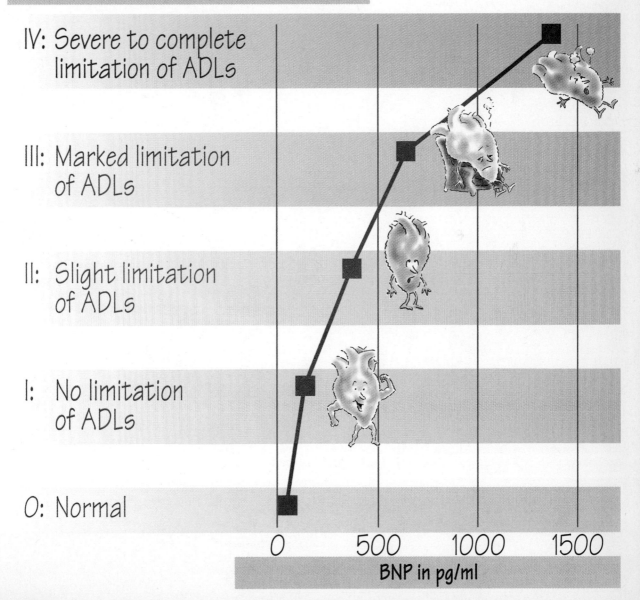

IV: Severe to complete limitation of ADLs

III: Marked limitation of ADLs

II: Slight limitation of ADLs

I: No limitation of ADLs

0: Normal

0   500   1000   1500

BNP in pg/ml

Tests for general screening

General screening tests are used to evaluate overall health and response to treatment.

Electrolyte tests

Electrolytes—which occur in the fluids both inside and outside cells—are crucial for nearly all cellular reactions and functions.

These electrolytes affect my rhythm.

Potassium, calcium, magnesium

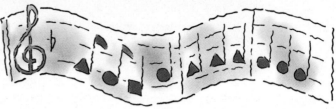

These electrolytes influence my fluid balance and acid-base status.

Sodium, chloride, carbon dioxide

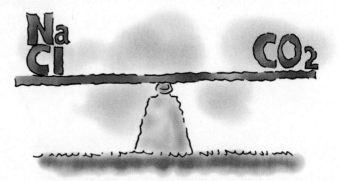

▲ Potassium

- Most critical value
- Has narrow therapeutic range
- Imbalances cause life-threatening arrhythmias
- Affected by diuretics, penicillin G, and low insulin

● Calcium

- High values cause cardiac toxicity and arrhythmias
- Elevations commonly caused by cancer or hyperparathyroidism

■ Magnesium

- High values cause ECG changes, ventricular tachycardia, and ventricular fibrillation
- Low values cause ECG changes, bradycardia, and hypotension

Sodium

- Maintains osmotic pressure, acid-base balance, and nerve impulse transmission
- Levels decreased in severe heart failure
- Decreased by diuretics, high triglycerides, and low blood protein

Chloride

- Partners with sodium to maintain fluid and acid-base balance
- Low levels in heart failure and metabolic acidosis

Carbon dioxide

- Primarily made up of bicarbonate
- Regulated by the kidneys
- Levels lowered by thiazide diuretics

memory board

The electrolytes most closely associated with cardiac status are magnesium, calcium, sodium, chloride, potassium, and carbon dioxide. To remember them, think "**M**y **C**at **S**ylvester **C**an **P**lay **C**ards."

Normal electrolyte values

- **M**agnesium: 1.3–2.1 mg/dl
- **C**alcium: 8.2–10.2 mg/dl
- **S**odium: 135–145 mEq/L
- **C**hloride: 100–108 mEq/L
- **P**otassium: 3.5–5 mEq/L
- **C**arbon dioxide: 23–30 mEq/L

Coagulation tests

Activated partial thromboplastin time (aPTT), prothrombin time (PT), bleeding time, and activated clotting time (ACT) are tests that measure clotting time. They're used to measure response to treatment as well as to screen for clotting disorders.

Understanding clotting

Clotting is initiated through two different pathways.

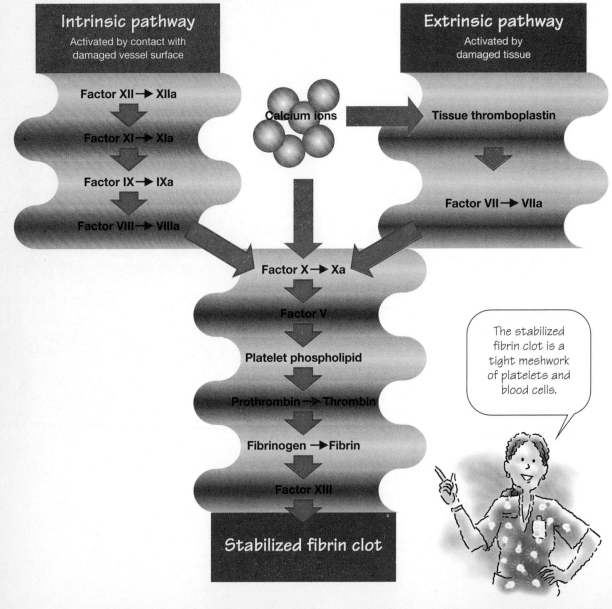

Common tests for clotting

Test	Action	Clinical uses	Where performed	Normal range	Therapeutic ranges	Panic value
ACT	Measures overall coagulation activity	♥ Evaluates effects of high dose heparin therapy during cardiac procedures	Bedside	70 to 120 seconds	2 times normal range	Unknown
Bleeding time	Determines platelet function abnormalities	♥ Screens for platelet abnormalities before or during surgery ♥ Used to diagnose von Willebrand's disease, vascular disorders, hemostatic dysfunctions	Bedside	3 to 10 minutes	Unknown	> 15 minutes
aPTT	Measures defects in intrinsic and common clotting pathways	♥ Evaluates effects of heparin therapy ♥ Assesses overall coagulation system	Laboratory	21 to 35 seconds	2 to 2.5 times normal range	> 70 seconds
PT	Directly measures deficits in extrinsic and common clotting pathways	♥ Evaluates effects of coumarin therapies ♥ Assesses for vitamin K deficiency ♥ Used to diagnose liver failure	Laboratory	11 to 13 seconds	2 to 2.5 times normal range	> 30 seconds

Understanding INR

Because PT measurements vary from laboratory to laboratory, International Normalized Ratio (INR) is generally viewed as the best standardized measurement of PT. Both are used for monitoring warfarin treatment. Guidelines for patients receiving warfarin therapy recommend an INR of 2.0 to 3.0, except for patients with mechanical prosthetic heart valves. For those patients, an INR of 2.5 to 3.5 is recommended.

What's the problem?

Increased INR values may indicate disseminated intravascular coagulation, cirrhosis, hepatitis, vitamin K deficiency, salicylate intoxication, or uncontrolled oral anticoagulation.

Electrocardiography

12-lead ECG

A commonly used diagnostic tool, the 12-lead ECG can help identify myocardial ischemia, MI, rhythm and conduction disturbances, chamber enlargement, electrolyte imbalances, and drug toxicity. The standard 12-lead ECG uses a series of electrodes placed on the patient's extremities and chest wall to assess the heart from 12 different views (leads).

> Six unipolar precordial leads (V_1 to V_6) show the heart from the **horizontal plane.**

> Three bipolar limb leads (I, II, and III) and three unipolar augmented limb leads (aV_R, aV_L, and aV_F) show the heart from the **frontal plane.**

Ground

Understanding ECG leads

ECG waveforms vary depending on the leads being viewed and the rhythm of the heart. To make an accurate assessment of the heart's electrical activity, an ECG needs to be evaluated from every view.

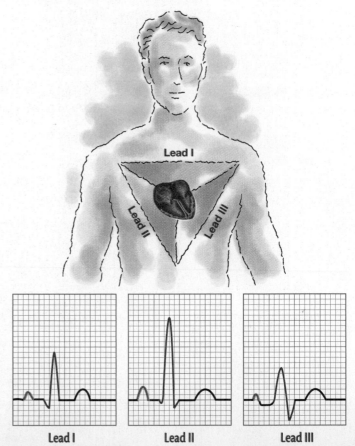

Lead I

Lead II

Lead III

Lead I   Lead II   Lead III

Locating myocardial damage with a 12-lead ECG

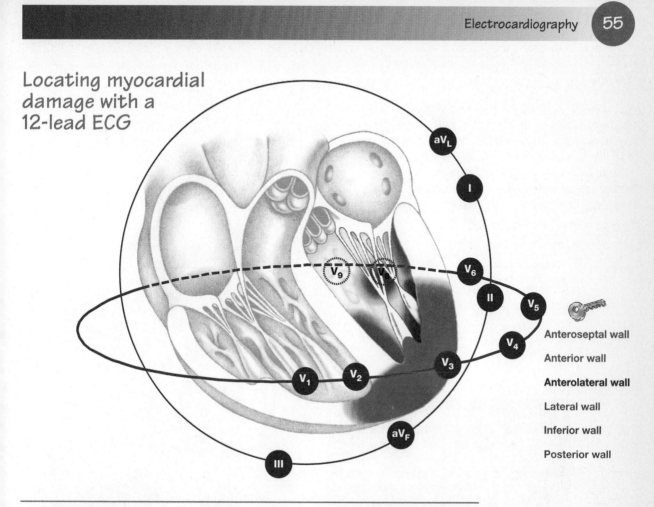

Anteroseptal wall

Anterior wall

Anterolateral wall

Lateral wall

Inferior wall

Posterior wall

Wall affected	Leads	Artery involved	Reciprocal changes
Anteroseptal	V_1, V_2, V_3, V_4	Left anterior descending (LAD)	None
Anterior	V_2, V_3, V_4	Left coronary artery, LAD	II, III, aV_F
Anterolateral	I, aV_L, V_3, V_4, V_5, V_6	LAD and diagonal branches, circumflex and marginal branches	II, III, aV_F
Lateral	I, aV_L, V_5, V_6	Circumflex branch of left coronary artery	II, III, aV_F
Inferior	II, III, aV_F	Right coronary artery (RCA)	I, aV_L
Posterior	V_8, V_9	RCA or circumflex	V_1, V_2, V_3, V_4 (R greater than S in V_1 and V_2, ST-segment depression, elevated T wave)

Exercise ECG

Exercise ECG, or *stress testing*, is a noninvasive procedure that helps assess the heart's response to an increased workload. Stop the test if the patient experiences chest pain, fatigue, severe dyspnea, claudication, weakness or dizziness, hypotension, pallor or vasoconstriction, disorientation, ataxia, ischemic ECG changes, rhythm disturbances or heart block, or ventricular conduction abnormalities.

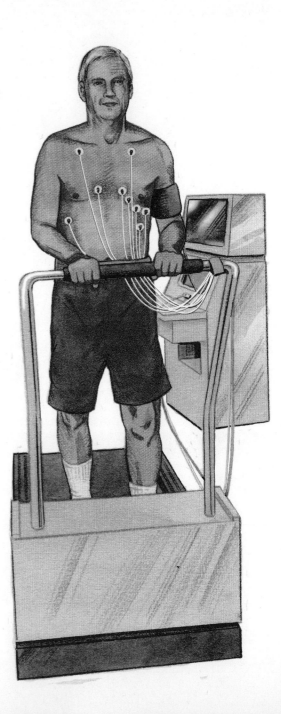

Drug-induced stress tests

If a patient can't tolerate physical activity, a drug (dipyridamole, adenosine, or dobutamine) can be administered to cause the heart to react as if the person were exercising. The drug is given I.V. along with thallium (a radioactive substance known as a *tracer*). Those areas of the heart muscle that lack adequate blood supply pick up the tracer very slowly, if at all.

A nuclear scanner records a set of images; a second set of images is taken 3 to 4 hours later. A cardiologist uses these images to determine areas of heart muscle with diminished blood supply or permanent damage from an MI.

Holter monitoring

Also called *ambulatory ECG*, Holter monitoring records the heart's activity as the patient follows his normal routine. The patient wears a small electronic recorder connected to electrodes placed on his chest and keeps a diary of his activities and associated symptoms. Used to identify intermittent arrhythmias, this test usually lasts about 24 hours.

A look at a Holter monitor

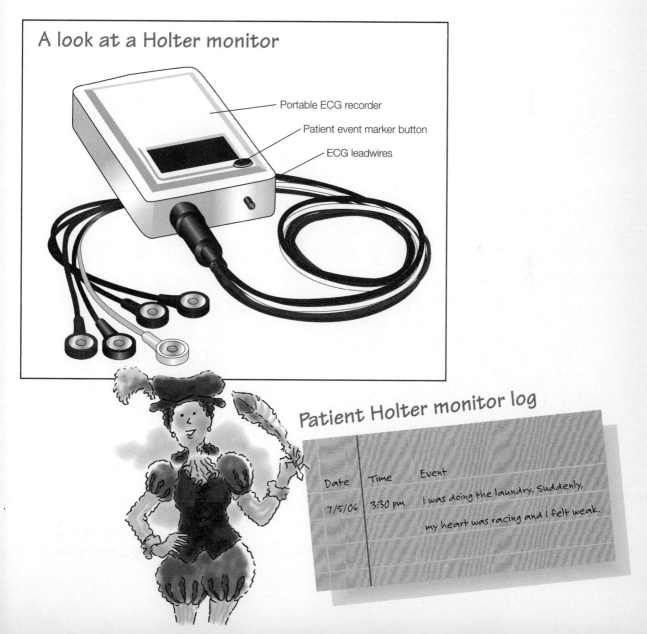

Portable ECG recorder

Patient event marker button

ECG leadwires

Patient Holter monitor log

Date	Time	Event
7/5/06	3:30 pm	I was doing the laundry. Suddenly, my heart was racing and I felt weak.

Electrophysiology studies

Electrophysiology studies are used to help determine the cause of an arrhythmia and the best treatment for it. A bipolar or tripolar electrode catheter is threaded into a vein, through the right atrium, and across the septal leaflet of the tricuspid valve. The heart's usual conduction is recorded first. The catheter sends electrical signals to the heart to change the heart rate and initiate an arrhythmia. Various drugs are then tried to terminate the arrhythmia.

The femoral vein is the most common choice for catheter insertion. However, the subclavian, internal jugular, or brachial vein may also be used.

Femoral vein

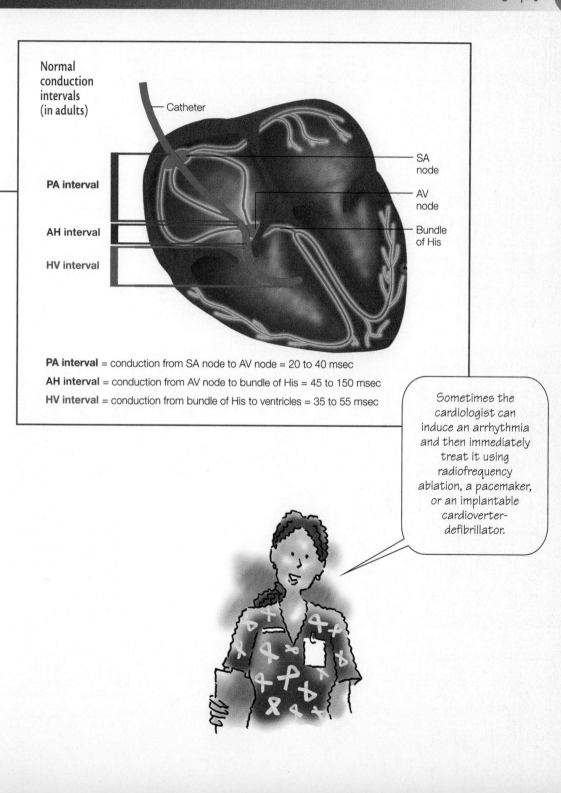

Normal
conduction
intervals
(in adults)

— Catheter

SA
node

AV
node

Bundle
of His

PA interval

AH interval

HV interval

PA interval = conduction from SA node to AV node = 20 to 40 msec

AH interval = conduction from AV node to bundle of His = 45 to 150 msec

HV interval = conduction from bundle of His to ventricles = 35 to 55 msec

Sometimes the cardiologist can induce an arrhythmia and then immediately treat it using radiofrequency ablation, a pacemaker, or an implantable cardioverter-defibrillator.

Imaging tests

Various imaging and radiographic tests are used to help visualize heart structures and blood vessels throughout the cardiovascular system. Although many of these tests are noninvasive and quick to perform, some require the insertion of a cardiac catheter, injection of a contrast medium, or nuclear medicine to further enhance the view.

Cardiac catheterization

Cardiac catheterization involves passing a catheter through veins and arteries to perform various measurements. It's used to:

- measure heart chamber and pulmonary artery pressures
- check blood flow between the heart chambers
- determine valve competence
- monitor cardiac wall contractility
- detect intracardiac shunts
- visualize the coronary arteries.

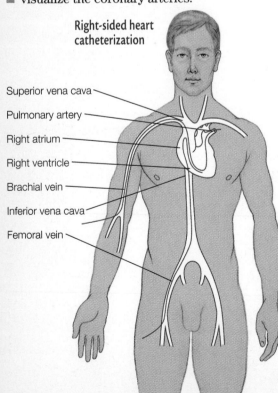

Right-sided heart catheterization

Superior vena cava
Pulmonary artery
Right atrium
Right ventricle
Brachial vein
Inferior vena cava
Femoral vein

Upper limits of normal pressure curves

Chambers of the right side of the heart

Two pressure complexes are represented for each chamber. Complexes at the far right in this diagram represent simultaneous recordings of pressures from the right atrium, right ventricle, and pulmonary artery.

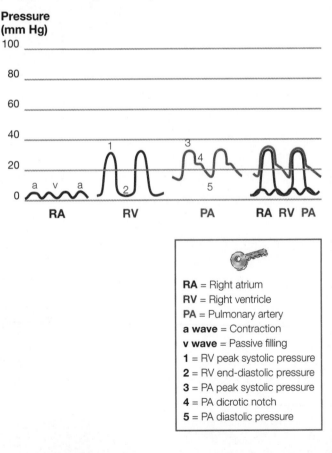

Pressure (mm Hg)

RA = Right atrium
RV = Right ventricle
PA = Pulmonary artery
a wave = Contraction
v wave = Passive filling
1 = RV peak systolic pressure
2 = RV end-diastolic pressure
3 = PA peak systolic pressure
4 = PA dicrotic notch
5 = PA diastolic pressure

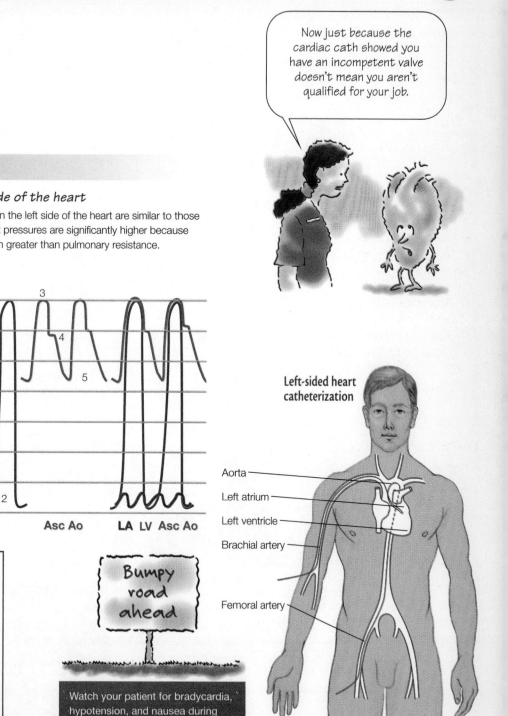

Now just because the cardiac cath showed you have an incompetent valve doesn't mean you aren't qualified for your job.

Chambers of the left side of the heart

Overall pressure configurations in the left side of the heart are similar to those of the right side of the heart, but pressures are significantly higher because systemic flow resistance is much greater than pulmonary resistance.

Pressure (mm Hg)

Left-sided heart catheterization

Aorta
Left atrium
Left ventricle
Brachial artery
Femoral artery

LA = Left atrium
LV = Left ventricle
Asc Ao = Ascending aorta
a wave = Contraction
v wave = Passive filling
1 = LV peak systolic pressure
2 = LV end-diastolic pressure
3 = PA peak systolic pressure
4 = PA dicrotic notch
5 = PA diastolic pressure

Bumpy road ahead

Watch your patient for bradycardia, hypotension, and nausea during femoral catheter removal.

Echocardiography

An echocardiograph uses ultrahigh-frequency sound waves to help examine the size, shape, and motion of the heart's structures. Here's how it works.

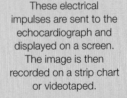

These electrical impulses are sent to the echocardiograph and displayed on a screen. The image is then recorded on a strip chart or videotaped.

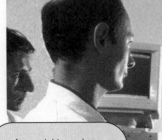

A special transducer is placed over an area on the chest where bone and lung tissues are absent. It directs sound waves to the heart structures and converts them to electrical impulses.

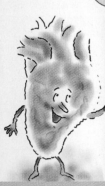

Picture this!

This computer graphic depicts an image of the heart's chambers and valves that's more detailed than an X-ray. The ultrasound waves that rebound (or echo) off the heart can show the size, shape, and movement of cardiac structures as well as the flow of blood through the heart, which helps analyze valvular function and heart pressures.

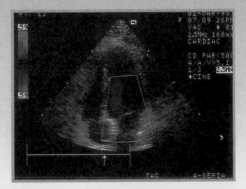

Comparing two types of echocardiography

The most commonly used echocardiographic techniques are M-mode (motion mode) and two-dimensional. In many cases, the techniques are performed together to complement each other. Echocardiography may be used to detect mitral stenosis, mitral valve prolapse, aortic insufficiency, wall motion abnormalities, and pericardial effusion. The shaded areas beneath the transducer identify cardiac structures that intercept and reflect the transducer's ultrasonic waves.

In M-mode echocardiography, a single, pencil-like ultrasound beam strikes the heart, producing an "ice pick," or vertical, view of cardiac structures. The echo tracings are plotted against time. This mode is especially useful for precisely viewing cardiac structures.

Transducer

Anterolateral chest wall

Right ventricular anterior wall

Right ventricle

Interventricular septum

Aortic valve

Left ventricle

Left atrium

Left ventricular posterior wall

In two-dimensional echocardiography, the ultrasound beam rapidly sweeps through a 30-degree arc, producing a cross-sectional, or fan-shaped, view of cardiac structures. Appearing as a real-time video display, this technique is useful for recording lateral motion and providing the correct spatial relationship between cardiac structures.

Road narrows

Ventricular wall motion changes on echocardiography before and after exercise stress testing can show myocardial ischemia.

It must
be TEE
time!

Transesophageal echocardiography

In transesophageal echocardiography (TEE), ultrasonography is combined with endoscopy to provide a better view of the heart's structures.

How it's done

A small transducer is attached to the end of a gastroscope and inserted into the esophagus so that images of the heart's structure can be taken from the posterior of the heart. This test causes less tissue penetration and interference from chest-wall structures and produces high-quality images of the thoracic aorta (except for the superior ascending aorta, which is shadowed by the trachea).

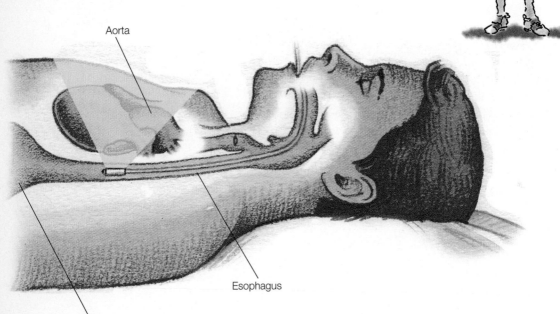

Aorta

Esophagus

Stomach

And why

TEE is used to evaluate valvular disease or repairs.
It's also used to diagnose:
- thoracic and aortic disorders
- endocarditis
- congenital heart disease
- intracardiac thrombi
- tumors.

> With TEE, I guess the old saying is true: The way to a man's heart is through his stomach...or at least through his esophagus!

memory board

Complications of TEE

Respiratory depression from sedation
Aspiration of secretions into trachea
Vasovagal reaction from vagus nerve stimulation
Esophageal perforation by transducer

> My notes say doctors **RAVE** about TEE!

Cardiac magnetic resonance imaging

Also known as *nuclear magnetic resonance*, cardiac magnetic resonance imaging (MRI) yields high-resolution, tomographic, three-dimensional images of the heart. Cardiac MRI permits visualization of valve leaflets and structures, pericardial abnormalities and processes, ventricular hypertrophy, cardiac neoplasm, infarcted tissue, anatomic malformations, and structural deformities. It can be used to monitor the progression of ischemic heart disease and the effectiveness of treatment.

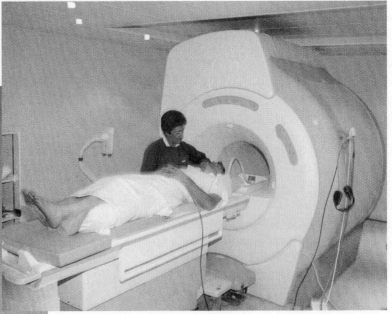

The MRI scanner records the electromagnetic signals the nuclei emit. The scanner then translates the signals into detailed pictures. The resulting images show tissue characteristics without lung or bone interference, as shown here.

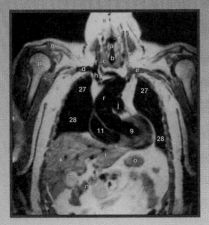

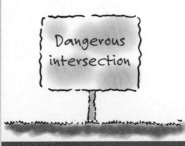

Dangerous intersection

Don't let your patients with pacemakers or implantable cardioverter-defibrillators in here; metal attracts!

Cardiac positron emission tomography

Cardiac positron emission tomography (PET) scanning combines elements of computed tomography scanning and conventional radionuclide imaging.

How it works

Radioisotopes are administered to the patient by injection, inhalation, or I.V. infusion. One isotope targets blood; one targets glucose.

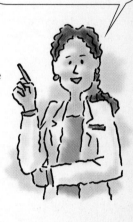

You can reassure your patient undergoing PET that he's getting no more radiation than a routine X-ray — but much better pictures.

These isotopes emit particles called *positrons*.

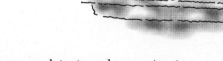

The PET scanner detects and reconstructs the positrons to form an image.

What it shows

■ Normal blood flow and glucose metabolism indicates good coronary perfusion.
■ Decreased blood flow with increased glucose metabolism indicates ischemia.
■ Decreased blood flow with decreased glucose metabolism shows necrotic or scarred heart tissue.

Cardiac blood pool imaging

Cardiac blood pool imaging (also called *multiple-gated acquisition [MUGA] scanning*) is used to evaluate regional and global ventricular performance.

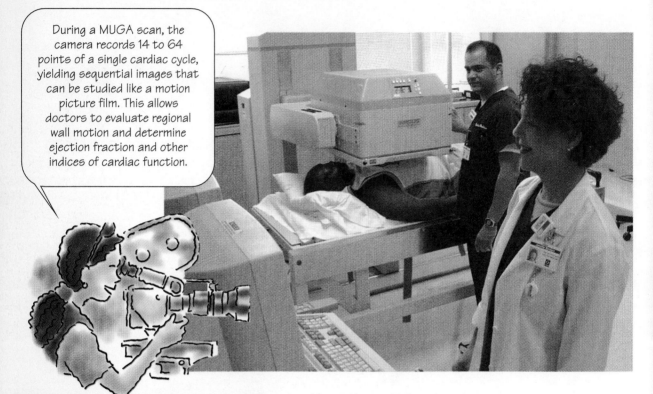

During a MUGA scan, the camera records 14 to 64 points of a single cardiac cycle, yielding sequential images that can be studied like a motion picture film. This allows doctors to evaluate regional wall motion and determine ejection fraction and other indices of cardiac function.

Varieties are the spice of life

Many variations of the MUGA scan are available:
■ In the *stress MUGA* test, the same test is performed at rest and after exercise to detect changes in ejection fraction and cardiac output.
■ In the *nitroglycerin MUGA* test, the scintillation camera records points in the cardiac cycle after the sublingual administration of nitroglycerin to assess the drug's effect on ventricular function.

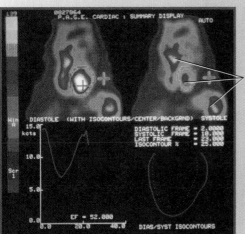

Blood flow

Did you know?

The MUGA scan is the most accurate way to measure ejection fraction? Oncologists use it to detect early signs of heart damage from cardiotoxic chemotherapeutic drugs such as adriamycin.

Hot and cold spot imaging

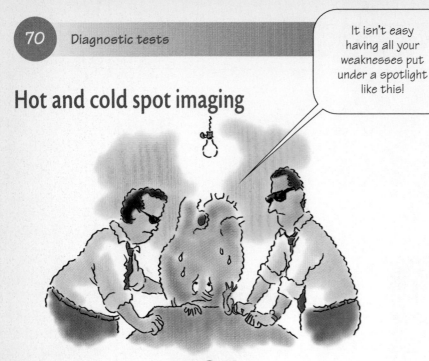

It isn't easy having all your weaknesses put under a spotlight like this!

$$^{99m}Tc + MI = \textbf{HOT}$$

Technetium-99m (^{99m}Tc) pyrophosphate scanning, also known as *hot spot imaging* or *PYP scanning*, helps diagnose acute myocardial injury by showing the location and size of newly damaged myocardial tissue.

How it works

■ ^{99m}Tc pyrophosphate is injected into the patient.
■ Isotopes are absorbed by damaged cells.
■ Damaged areas show as orange to bright red spots on the image.
■ The scan reveals transmural, right ventricular, and posterior infarctions.
■ Ventricular aneurysms and tumors are also visible.

Test tip

Tell your patient to expect to lie on his back with his arms above his head during and up to 30 minutes after the test. This allows the scanner to move 360 degrees around his body.

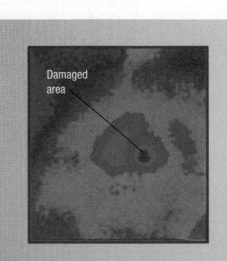

Damaged area

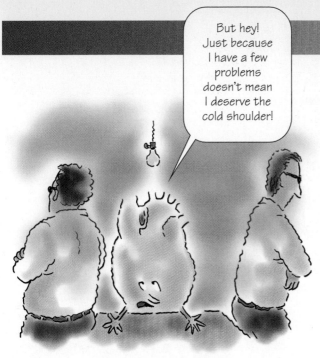

> But hey! Just because I have a few problems doesn't mean I deserve the cold shoulder!

Tl^{201} + MI = COLD

Also known as *cold spot imaging*, thallium (Tl^{201}) scanning evaluates myocardial blood flow and myocardial cell status.

How it works

■ Tl^{201} is injected into the patient.

■ Isotopes are rapidly absorbed by healthy heart tissue and emit gamma rays. Unhealthy tissue slowly absorbs isotopes.

■ Damaged areas show as dark blue to purple spots on the image.

■ The scan reveals ischemic and infarcted areas.

■ The test is also used to evaluate ventricular function and the presence of pericardial effusion.

Test tip

If your patient can't raise his arms, one-dimensional Tl^{201} scanning can still be done. Pictures are taken from three different views (called *planar imaging*).

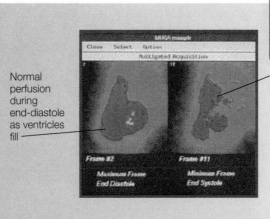

Normal perfusion during end-diastole as ventricles fill

Normal perfusion during end-systole as ventricles contract

Doppler ultrasonography

Doppler ultrasonography involves the use of high-frequency sound waves to evaluate blood flow in the major vessels of the trunk (heart and intra-abdominal organs) and extremities (arms and legs) and in the extracranial cerebrovascular system (neck). This noninvasive test shows the direction and speed of blood flow and can detect turbulent flow due to narrowing or blockage of blood vessels.

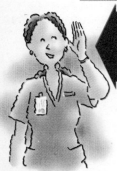

> Measurement of systolic pressure with a Doppler transducer helps detect the presence, location, and extent of peripheral arterial occlusive disease.

A handheld transducer directs high-frequency sound waves to the artery or vein being tested.

The sound waves strike moving RBCs.

The transducer then amplifies the sound waves to permit direct listening and graphic recording of blood flow.

The sound waves are reflected back to the transducer at frequencies that correspond to blood flow velocity through the vessel.

Listen up!

Pulse volume recorder testing may be performed along with Doppler ultrasonography to yield a quantitative recording of changes in blood volume or flow in an extremity or organ.

Normally, venous blood flow fluctuates with respiration, so observing changes in sound wave frequency during respiration helps detect venous occlusive disease. Compression maneuvers can also help detect occlusion of the veins as well as occlusion or stenosis of carotid arteries. Abnormal images (seen on duplex ultrasonography) and Doppler signals may indicate plaque, stenosis, occlusion, dissection, aneurysm, carotid body tumor, and arteritis.

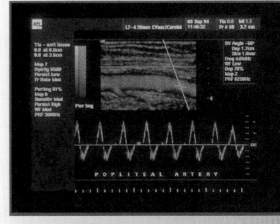

Doppler of popliteal artery

Color flow duplex image of popliteal artery with normal triphasic Doppler flow.

Measuring the ankle-brachial index

A Doppler ultrasound device can also be used to measure ankle-brachial index (ABI) to help identify peripheral vascular disease. To perform this test, follow these steps.

1 Explain the procedure to the patient.

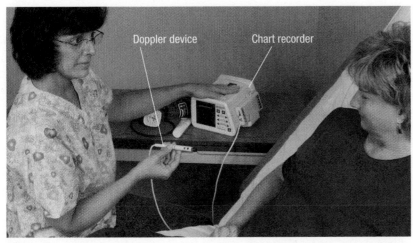

Doppler device   Chart recorder

2 Gather your materials.

3 Wash your hands.

4 Apply warm conductivity gel to the patient's arm where the brachial pulse has been palpated and then obtain the systolic reading.

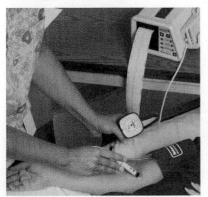

5 Locate the posterior tibial pulse and repeat the procedure, recording your reading.

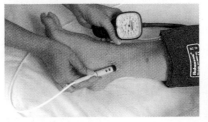

6 Locate the dorsalis pedis pulse and repeat the procedure.

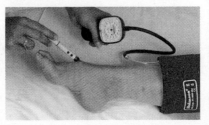

7 Use the chart below to calculate the ABI. Document your findings.

Calculating ABI

To calculate ABI, divide the higher systolic pressure obtained for each leg (dorsalis pedia or posterior tibial) by the higher brachial systolic pressure.

Sample systolic readings (mm Hg)	Left	Right
Posterior tibial	128	96
Dorsalis pedis	130	90
Brachial	132	130
Calculations	130 ÷ 132 = 0.98	96 ÷ 132 = 0.73

What the results mean

■ **Greater than 1.3:** Unreliable and inconclusive; possibly false-high readings produced by calcified vessels (such as occurs in diabetes)
■ **1.01 to 1.3:** Correlates with patient history (especially in diabetes)
■ **0.97 to 1:** Normal
■ **0.8 to 0.96:** Mild ischemia
■ **0.4 to 0.79:** Moderate to severe ischemia
■ **0.39 or less:** Severe ischemia; danger of limb loss

Venography

Also known as *ascending contrast phlebography*, venography is radiographic examination of veins in a lower extremity. During this test, a catheter is inserted into a vein (usually through the foot) and a contrast medium is injected. X-rays are then used to visualize the internal structures.

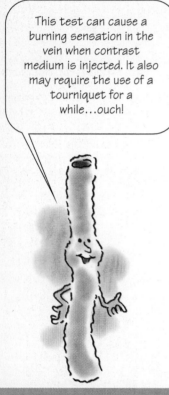

This test can cause a burning sensation in the vein when contrast medium is injected. It also may require the use of a tourniquet for a while…ouch!

What's the problem?

This procedure isn't used for routine screening because it exposes the patient to relatively high doses of radiation and can cause such complications as phlebitis, local tissue damage and, occasionally, deep vein thrombosis. It's used in patients whose duplex ultrasound findings are unclear.

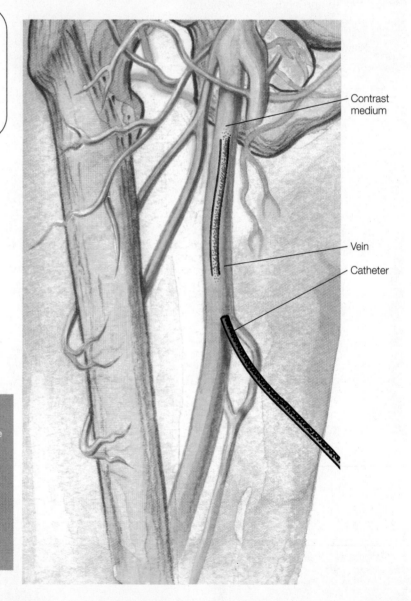

Contrast medium

Vein

Catheter

Peripheral arteriography

Peripheral arteriography, or *angiography,* is the injection of a contrast medium into the peripheral arteries accompanied by cineangiograms (rapidly changing movies on an intensified fluoroscopic screen), which record passage of the contrast medium through the vascular system. Arteriography can also be done using a magnetic resonance scanner and contrast medium.

Arteriography demonstrates the type (thrombus or embolus), location, and degree of obstruction, and collateral circulation. This procedure is particularly useful in chronic disease or for evaluating candidates for reconstructive surgery.

Angiograph of the femoral artery and its branches

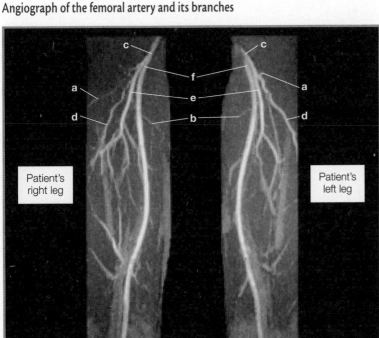

Patient's right leg

Patient's left leg

Be aware of the risks of injecting a contrast medium. Your patient may experience an allergic reaction to the dye, local tissue damage, bleeding or clotting at the puncture site, or even a stroke.

a = Lateral circumflex femoral artery
b = Medial circumflex femoral artery
c = Femoral artery
d = Descending branch of the profunda femoris artery
e = Profunda femoris artery
f = Femoral artery

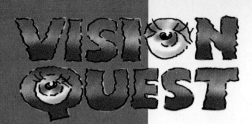

Matchmaker

Match the diagnostic test with its proper description.

1. BNP test ___

2. Echocardiography ___

3. Venography ___

4. Lipoprotein fractionation ___

5. MUGA scanning ___

6. aPTT ___

7. 12-lead ECG ___

A. Also known as *cardiac blood pool imaging*

B. Uses ultrahigh-frequency sound waves that bounce off cardiac structures

C. Isolates and measures three types of cholesterol in blood

D. Requires using a series of electrodes to view heart from different angles

E. Helps diagnose and grade the severity of heart failure based on hormone levels

F. Evaluates clotting factors and helps monitor response to heparin

G. Involves catheterization of lower extremity to view veins

"X" marks the spot

Place an "X" on this illustration over the area that represents myocardial damage.

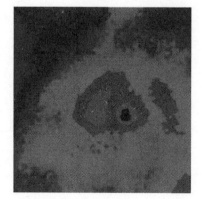

4 ECG interpretation

I'm the star of this show. Do you dig my rhythm?

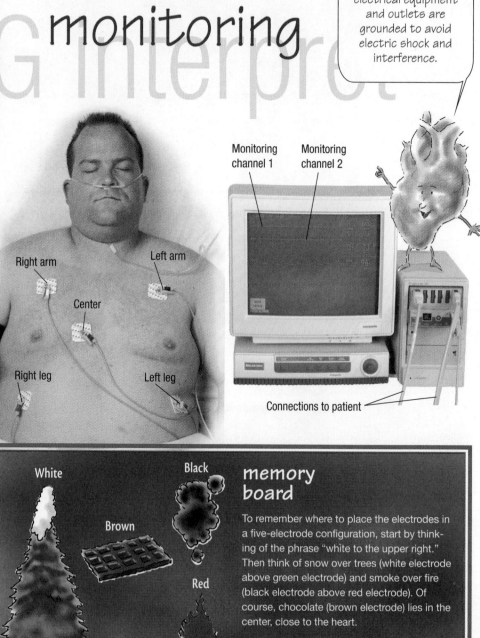

Cardiac monitoring

Make sure that all electrical equipment and outlets are grounded to avoid electric shock and interference.

Electrocardiography is used to diagnose and monitor cardiac disorders. When a patient is hospitalized, the first step is to begin continuous cardiac monitoring. In a hardwire system, the patient is connected directly to an electrocardiograph (ECG) by electrodes, leadwires, and a monitor cable. Most monitoring systems use three or five leads and provide a continuous readout of one or more leads simultaneously. Lead selection is based on the patient's clinical situation. Lead V_1 or V_6 and an appropriate limb lead are usually used.

Right arm

Left arm

Center

Right leg

Left leg

Monitoring channel 1

Monitoring channel 2

Connections to patient

memory board

White

Black

Brown

Red

To remember where to place the electrodes in a five-electrode configuration, start by thinking of the phrase "white to the upper right." Then think of snow over trees (white electrode above green electrode) and smoke over fire (black electrode above red electrode). Of course, chocolate (brown electrode) lies in the center, close to the heart.

Leading leads

These illustrations show the heart views obtained by various leads as well as the best uses for each lead. Current moving from negative to positive gives an upward deflection of the complexes on the ECG; current moving from positive to negative gives a downward deflection.

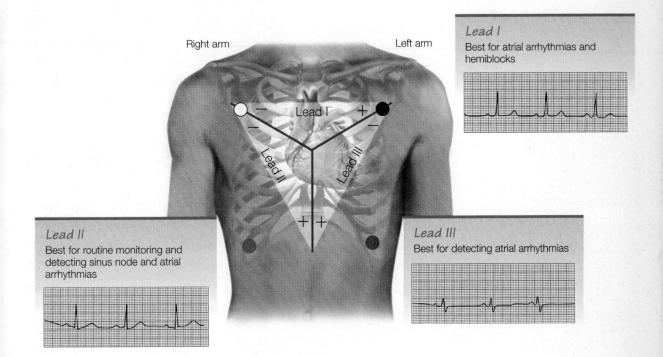

Right arm   Left arm

Lead I

Lead II

Lead III

Lead I
Best for atrial arrhythmias and hemiblocks

Lead II
Best for routine monitoring and detecting sinus node and atrial arrhythmias

Lead III
Best for detecting atrial arrhythmias

Viewing V_6 requires moving the chest lead from the V_1 precordial position to the V_6 precordial position.

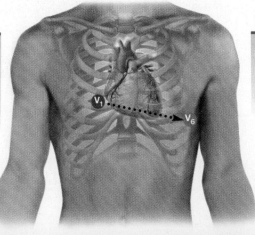

Lead V_1
Best for P wave changes, QRS complex arrhythmias, and tachycardia

Lead V_6
Best for ventricular conduction changes

Troubleshooting monitor problems

What you see	What might cause it	What to do about it
Artifact (waveform interference)	▪ Seizures	▪ If the patient is having a seizure, notify the doctor and intervene as ordered.
	▪ Chills	▪ Keep the patient warm.
	▪ Anxiety	▪ Encourage him to relax.
	▪ Improper electrode application	▪ Check the electrodes and reapply them if needed. Clean the skin well. ▪ Check the electrode gel. If the gel is dry, apply new electrodes.
	▪ Short circuit in lead-wires or cable	▪ Replace broken equipment.
	▪ Electrical interference from other electrical equipment in the room	▪ Make sure all electrical equipment is attached to a common ground. ▪ Notify the biomedical department.
False high-rate alarm	▪ Gain setting too high, particularly with MCL_1 setting	▪ Assess the patient for signs and symptoms of hyperkalemia. ▪ Decrease gain.
Weak signals	▪ Improper electrode application	▪ Reapply the electrodes.
	▪ QRS complex too small to register	▪ Reset gain so that the height of the complex is greater than 1 mV. ▪ Try monitoring the patient on another lead.
	▪ Wire or cable failure	▪ Replace any faulty wires or cables.

What you see	What might cause it	What to do about it
Wandering baseline 	▪ Patient restlessness ▪ Improper electrode application; electrode positioned over bone	▪ Encourage the patient to relax. ▪ Reposition improperly placed electrodes.
Fuzzy baseline (electrical interference) 	▪ Electrical interference from other equipment in the room ▪ Improper grounding of the patient's bed ▪ Electrode malfunction	▪ Ensure that all electrical equipment is attached to a common ground. ▪ Ensure that the bed ground is attached to the room's common ground. ▪ Replace the electrodes.
Baseline (no waveform) 	▪ Improper electrode placement (perpendicular to axis of heart) ▪ Disconnected electrode ▪ Dry electrode gel ▪ Wire or cable failure	▪ Reposition improperly placed electrodes. ▪ Check if electrodes are disconnected. Reapply them as necessary. ▪ Check electrode gel. If the gel is dry, apply new electrodes. ▪ Replace faulty wires or cables.

Remember to treat the patient, not the monitor.

Rhythm strips

In electrocardiography, the electrical activity of the heart is displayed on a monitoring screen and can be printed onto a rhythm strip.

Worth the paper it's printed on

ECG paper consists of horizontal and vertical lines that form a grid.

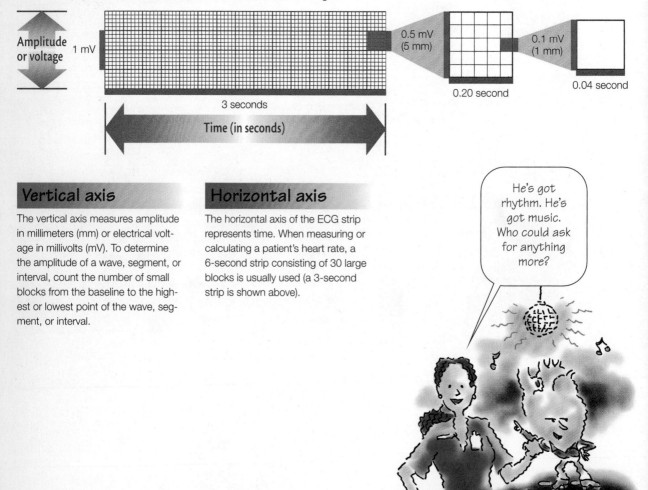

Amplitude or voltage
1 mV

0.5 mV (5 mm)

0.1 mV (1 mm)

0.20 second

0.04 second

3 seconds

Time (in seconds)

Vertical axis

The vertical axis measures amplitude in millimeters (mm) or electrical voltage in millivolts (mV). To determine the amplitude of a wave, segment, or interval, count the number of small blocks from the baseline to the highest or lowest point of the wave, segment, or interval.

Horizontal axis

The horizontal axis of the ECG strip represents time. When measuring or calculating a patient's heart rate, a 6-second strip consisting of 30 large blocks is usually used (a 3-second strip is shown above).

He's got rhythm. He's got music. Who could ask for anything more?

ECG components

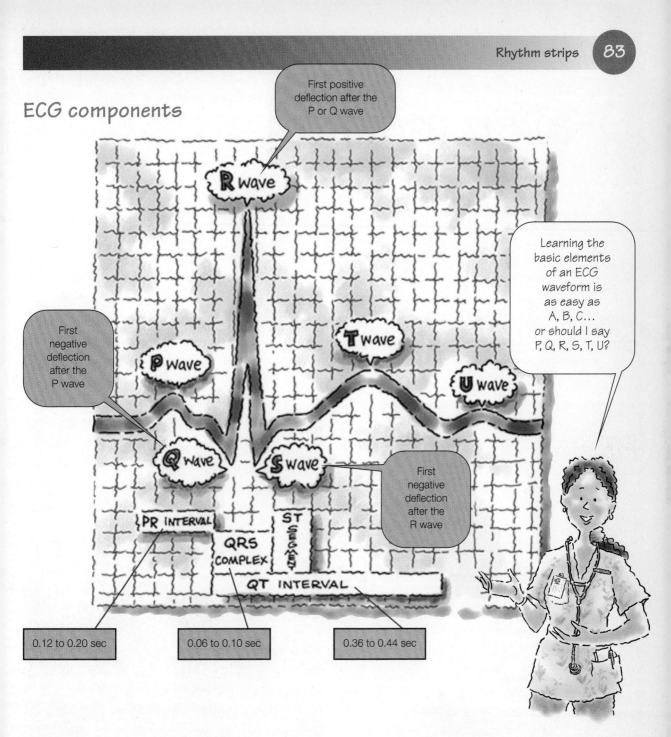

8-step method

1 Evaluate atrial and ventricular rhythms

For the atrial rhythm, use a pair of calipers to measure the interval between P waves (P-P interval) in several ECG cycles. Set the calipers at the same point—at the beginning of the wave or on its peak. The P wave should occur at regular intervals, with only small variations associated with respiration.

To check the ventricular rhythm, use calipers to measure the R-R intervals. Remember to place the calipers on the same point of the QRS complex. If the R-R intervals remain consistent, the ventricular rhythm is regular.

3 Evaluate the P wave

Observe the P wave's size, shape, and location in the waveform. If each QRS complex has a P wave, the sinoatrial (SA) node is initiating the electrical impulse, as it should be.

When using calipers to evaluate atrial rhythm, don't lift the calipers. Instead, rotate one of its legs to the next P wave to ensure accurate measurements.

2 Determine atrial and ventricular rates

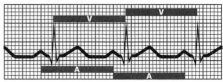

To determine the atrial rate when the heart rate is regular, count the number of small squares between identical points on two consecutive P waves, and then divide 1,500 by that number. To determine the ventricular rate, use the same method with two consecutive R waves.

Calculating rates

Three methods can be used to calculate the atrial or ventricular rate.

Times-10 method

The times-10 method is the quickest and best way to calculate the rate of an irregular rhythm. However, it can provide misleading numbers when the rate is very slow.

1,500 method

The 1,500 method, described above in step 2, is the most accurate method for regular rhythms, but it takes a little longer to calculate. First, count the number of small squares between two consecutive P waves using either the apex of the wave or the initial upstroke of the wave. Then divide 1,500 by that number to get the atrial rate. You can use the same method with two consecutive R waves to calculate the ventricular rate.

Sequence method

The sequence method is also only accurate at estimating regular rhythms. First, find a P wave that peaks on a heavy black line. Assign the following numbers to the next six heavy black lines: 300, 150, 100, 75, 60, and 50. Then find the next P wave peak. Estimate the rate based on the number assigned to the nearest heavy black line.

4 Calculate the PR interval

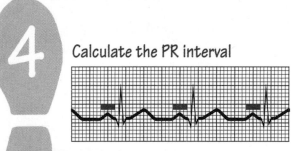

Count the number of small squares between the beginning of the P wave and the beginning of the QRS complex. Multiply the number of squares by 0.04 second. The normal interval is between 0.12 and 0.2 second, or between 3 and 5 small squares.

5 Calculate the duration of the QRS complex

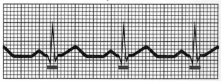

Count the number of squares between the beginning and the end of the QRS complex and multiply that number by 0.04 second. A normal QRS complex is less than 0.12 second, or less than 3 small squares wide. Some references specify 0.06 to 0.10 second as the normal duration of the QRS complex. Check to see if all QRS complexes are the same size and shape, and note if a complex appears after every P wave.

6 Evaluate the T wave

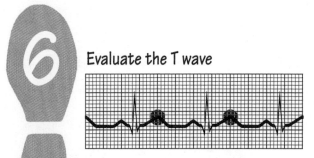

Check that T waves are present and have a normal shape, normal amplitude, and the same deflection as QRS complexes. Consider whether a P wave could be hidden in a T wave by looking for extra bumps in the waveform.

7 Calculate the duration of the QT interval

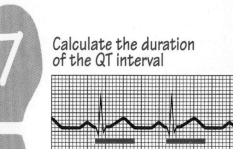

Count the number of squares from the beginning of the QRS complex to the end of the T wave. Multiply this number by 0.04 second. The normal range is 0.36 to 0.44 second, or 9 to 11 small squares wide.

8 Evaluate other components

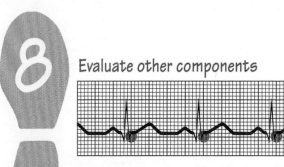

Quickly look for ectopic beats, aberrantly conducted beats, or other abnormalities. Then make sure the waveform doesn't reflect problems with the monitor. Next, check the ST segment for abnormalities and look for a U wave. Finally, classify the rhythm strip according to site of rhythm origin, rate, and rhythm.

Arrhythmias

Cardiac arrhythmias are variations in the normal pattern of electrical stimulation of the heart. Arrhythmias range from mild, causing no symptoms and requiring no treatment (such as sinus arrhythmia), to those that require emergency intervention and may cause death (such as ventricular fibrillation).

Arrhythmia locations

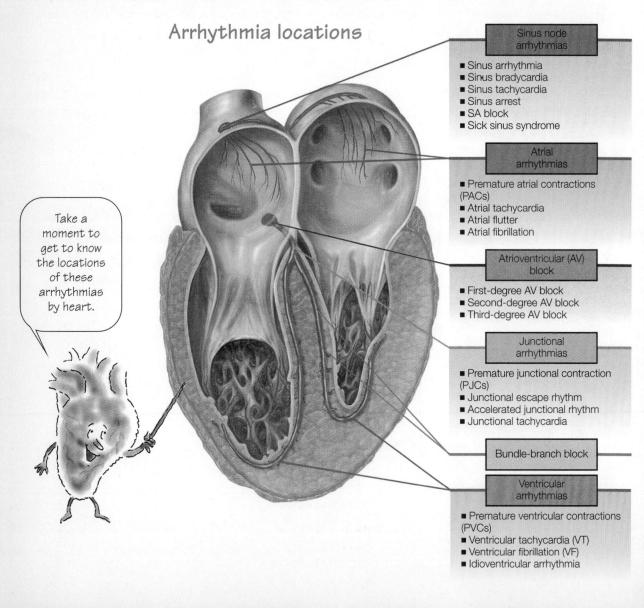

Take a moment to get to know the locations of these arrhythmias by heart.

Sinus node arrhythmias
- Sinus arrhythmia
- Sinus bradycardia
- Sinus tachycardia
- Sinus arrest
- SA block
- Sick sinus syndrome

Atrial arrhythmias
- Premature atrial contractions (PACs)
- Atrial tachycardia
- Atrial flutter
- Atrial fibrillation

Atrioventricular (AV) block
- First-degree AV block
- Second-degree AV block
- Third-degree AV block

Junctional arrhythmias
- Premature junctional contraction (PJCs)
- Junctional escape rhythm
- Accelerated junctional rhythm
- Junctional tachycardia

Bundle-branch block

Ventricular arrhythmias
- Premature ventricular contractions (PVCs)
- Ventricular tachycardia (VT)
- Ventricular fibrillation (VF)
- Idioventricular arrhythmia

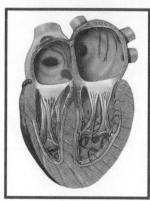

Sinus node arrhythmias

When the heart functions normally, the SA node, also called the *sinus node*, acts as the primary pacemaker. The SA node assumes this role because its automatic firing rate (60 to 100 beats/minute in an adult at rest) exceeds that of the heart's other pacemakers. Sinus node arrhythmias occur when the node's firing rate increases or decreases.

Pacemaker rates

PACEMAKER	RATE (BEATS/MINUTE)
SA node	60 to 100
AV node	40 to 60
Purkinje fibers	20 to 40

Sinus arrhythmia

In sinus arrhythmia, the SA node fires irregularly. When sinus arrhythmia is related to respirations, heart rate increases with inspiration and decreases with expiration, as shown at right. Sinus arrhythmia may be caused by inferior-wall myocardial infarction (MI), use of digoxin (Lanoxin) or morphine (Roxanol), and increased intracranial pressure. If sinus arrhythmia is unrelated to respiration, the underlying cause may require treatment.

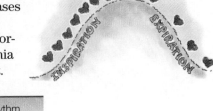

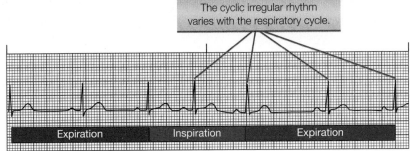

The cyclic irregular rhythm varies with the respiratory cycle.

Expiration   Inspiration   Expiration

Rhythm
- Irregular
- Corresponds to the respiratory cycle
- P-P interval and R-R interval shorter during respiratory inspiration; longer during expiration
- Difference between longest and shortest P-P interval exceeds 0.12 second

Rate
- Usually within normal limits (60 to 100 beats/minute)
- Varies with respiration (increases during inspiration; decreases during expiration)

P wave
- Normal size
- Normal configuration
- P wave before each QRS complex

PR interval
- May vary slightly
- Within normal limits

QRS complex
- Preceded by P wave

T wave
- Normal size
- Normal configuration

QT interval
- May vary slightly
- Usually within normal limits

Other
- Phasic slowing and quickening

Sinus bradycardia

Sinus bradycardia is a heart rate less than 60 beats/minute. If the rate falls below 45 beats/minute, patients usually have signs and symptoms of decreased cardiac output, such as hypotension, dizziness, confusion and, possibly, syncope.

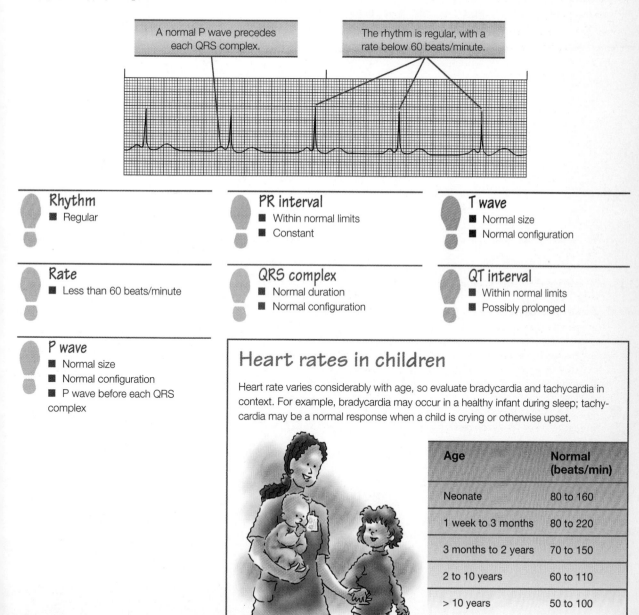

A normal P wave precedes each QRS complex.

The rhythm is regular, with a rate below 60 beats/minute.

Rhythm
- Regular

Rate
- Less than 60 beats/minute

P wave
- Normal size
- Normal configuration
- P wave before each QRS complex

PR interval
- Within normal limits
- Constant

QRS complex
- Normal duration
- Normal configuration

T wave
- Normal size
- Normal configuration

QT interval
- Within normal limits
- Possibly prolonged

Heart rates in children

Heart rate varies considerably with age, so evaluate bradycardia and tachycardia in context. For example, bradycardia may occur in a healthy infant during sleep; tachycardia may be a normal response when a child is crying or otherwise upset.

Age	Normal (beats/min)
Neonate	80 to 160
1 week to 3 months	80 to 220
3 months to 2 years	70 to 150
2 to 10 years	60 to 110
> 10 years	50 to 100

Sinus tachycardia

Sinus tachycardia in an adult is characterized by a sinus rate greater than 100 beats/minute. The rate rarely exceeds 180 beats/minute, except during strenuous exercise.

Sinus tachycardia in a patient who has had an acute MI suggests massive heart damage. Persistent tachycardia may signal impending heart failure or cardiogenic shock.

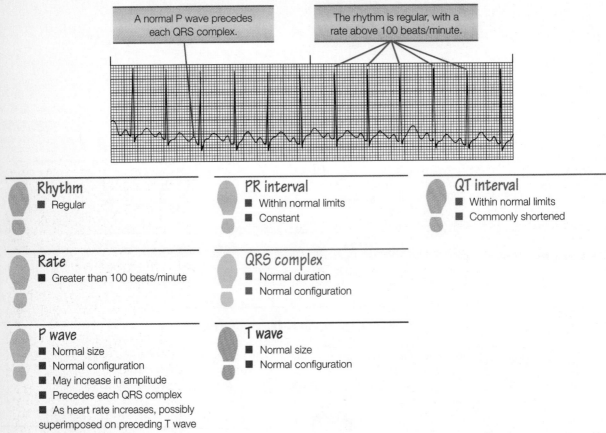

A normal P wave precedes each QRS complex.

The rhythm is regular, with a rate above 100 beats/minute.

Rhythm
- Regular

PR interval
- Within normal limits
- Constant

QT interval
- Within normal limits
- Commonly shortened

Rate
- Greater than 100 beats/minute

QRS complex
- Normal duration
- Normal configuration

P wave
- Normal size
- Normal configuration
- May increase in amplitude
- Precedes each QRS complex
- As heart rate increases, possibly superimposed on preceding T wave and difficult to identify

T wave
- Normal size
- Normal configuration

Sinus arrest

Atrial standstill occurs when the atria aren't stimulated and an entire PQRST complex is missing from an otherwise normal ECG strip. Atrial standstill is called *sinus pause* if one or two beats aren't formed and *sinus arrest* when three or more beats aren't formed. Causes of sinus arrest include acute infection, heart disease, use of some drugs, and vagal stimulation.

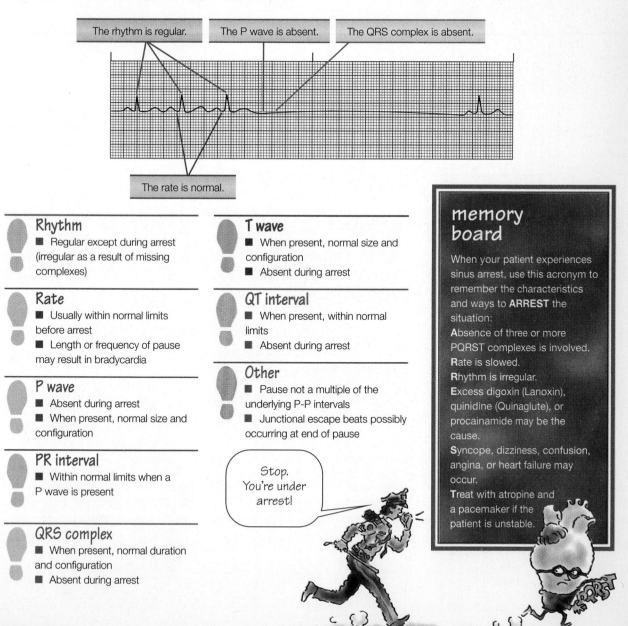

The rhythm is regular.

The P wave is absent.

The QRS complex is absent.

The rate is normal.

Rhythm
■ Regular except during arrest (irregular as a result of missing complexes)

Rate
■ Usually within normal limits before arrest
■ Length or frequency of pause may result in bradycardia

P wave
■ Absent during arrest
■ When present, normal size and configuration

PR interval
■ Within normal limits when a P wave is present

QRS complex
■ When present, normal duration and configuration
■ Absent during arrest

T wave
■ When present, normal size and configuration
■ Absent during arrest

QT interval
■ When present, within normal limits
■ Absent during arrest

Other
■ Pause not a multiple of the underlying P-P intervals
■ Junctional escape beats possibly occurring at end of pause

Stop. You're under arrest!

memory board

When your patient experiences sinus arrest, use this acronym to remember the characteristics and ways to **ARREST** the situation:
Absence of three or more PQRST complexes is involved.
Rate is slowed.
Rhythm is irregular.
Excess digoxin (Lanoxin), quinidine (Quinaglute), or procainamide may be the cause.
Syncope, dizziness, confusion, angina, or heart failure may occur.
Treat with atropine and a pacemaker if the patient is unstable.

SA block

In SA block, the SA node discharges impulses at regular intervals, but some of those impulses are delayed on the way to the atria. The most common block is the *SA exit block*. SA block may result from acute infection, an inferior-wall MI, coronary artery disease (CAD), hypertensive heart disease, sinus node disease, or use of medications, such as beta-adrenergic blockers, calcium channel blockers, inotropics, or antiarrhythmics.

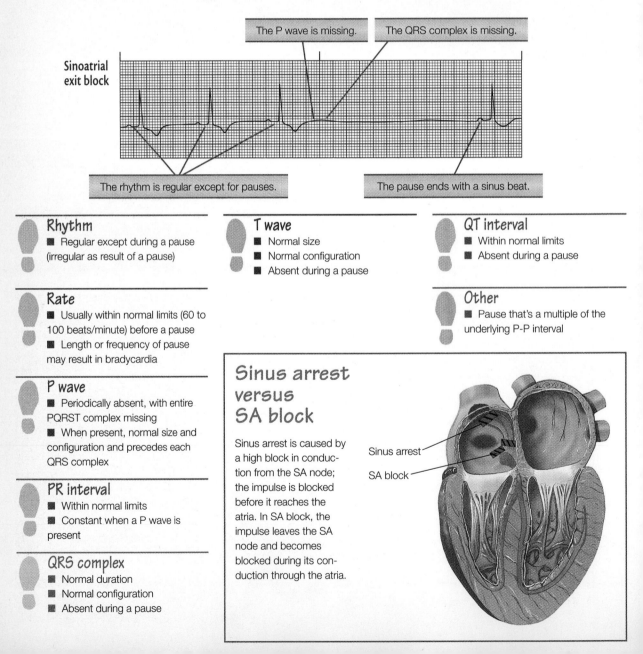

Sinoatrial exit block

The P wave is missing.

The QRS complex is missing.

The rhythm is regular except for pauses.

The pause ends with a sinus beat.

Rhythm
- Regular except during a pause (irregular as result of a pause)

Rate
- Usually within normal limits (60 to 100 beats/minute) before a pause
- Length or frequency of pause may result in bradycardia

P wave
- Periodically absent, with entire PQRST complex missing
- When present, normal size and configuration and precedes each QRS complex

PR interval
- Within normal limits
- Constant when a P wave is present

QRS complex
- Normal duration
- Normal configuration
- Absent during a pause

T wave
- Normal size
- Normal configuration
- Absent during a pause

QT interval
- Within normal limits
- Absent during a pause

Other
- Pause that's a multiple of the underlying P-P interval

Sinus arrest versus SA block

Sinus arrest is caused by a high block in conduction from the SA node; the impulse is blocked before it reaches the atria. In SA block, the impulse leaves the SA node and becomes blocked during its conduction through the atria.

Sinus arrest

SA block

Sick sinus syndrome

Also called *sinus nodal dysfunction*, sick sinus syndrome results either from a dysfunction of the sinus node's automaticity or from abnormal conduction or blockages of impulses coming out of the nodal region, including one or a combination of the following conditions:
- sinus bradycardia
- SA block
- sinus arrest
- sinus bradycardia alternating with sinus tachycardia
- episodes of atrial tachyarrhythmias, such as atrial fibrillation and atrial flutter
- failure of the sinus node to increase the heart rate with exercise.

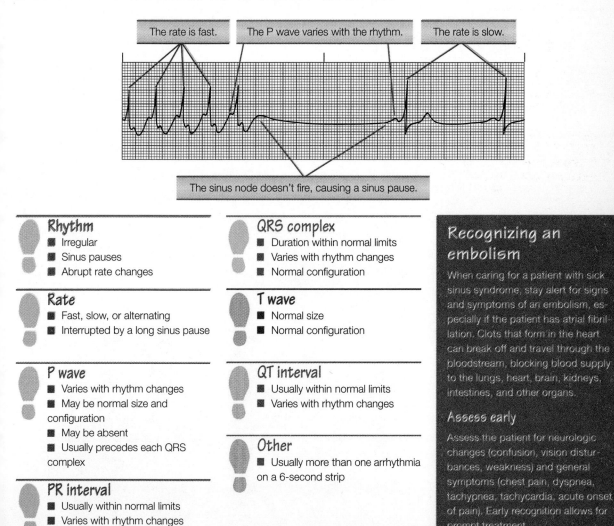

The rate is fast.

The P wave varies with the rhythm.

The rate is slow.

The sinus node doesn't fire, causing a sinus pause.

Rhythm
- Irregular
- Sinus pauses
- Abrupt rate changes

Rate
- Fast, slow, or alternating
- Interrupted by a long sinus pause

P wave
- Varies with rhythm changes
- May be normal size and configuration
- May be absent
- Usually precedes each QRS complex

PR interval
- Usually within normal limits
- Varies with rhythm changes

QRS complex
- Duration within normal limits
- Varies with rhythm changes
- Normal configuration

T wave
- Normal size
- Normal configuration

QT interval
- Usually within normal limits
- Varies with rhythm changes

Other
- Usually more than one arrhythmia on a 6-second strip

Recognizing an embolism

When caring for a patient with sick sinus syndrome, stay alert for signs and symptoms of an embolism, especially if the patient has atrial fibrillation. Clots that form in the heart can break off and travel through the bloodstream, blocking blood supply to the lungs, heart, brain, kidneys, intestines, and other organs.

Assess early

Assess the patient for neurologic changes (confusion, vision disturbances, weakness) and general symptoms (chest pain, dyspnea, tachypnea, tachycardia, acute onset of pain). Early recognition allows for prompt treatment.

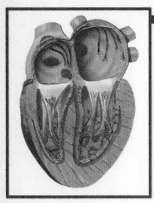

Atrial arrhythmias

The most common cardiac rhythm disturbances, atrial arrhythmias result from impulses originating in areas outside the SA node. They can affect ventricular filling time and diminish the strength of atrial kick (the contraction that normally provides the ventricles with about 30% of their blood).

Mechanisms of atrial arrhythmias

Mechanism	Characteristics	Possible causes
Altered automaticity	♥ Ability of atrial cardiac cells to initiate impulses on their own increases, triggering abnormal impulses.	♥ Hypoxia ♥ Hypocalcemia ♥ Digoxin (Lanoxin) toxicity ♥ Conditions that diminish sinoatrial node function
Reentry	♥ A slow conduction pathway delays impulse. ♥ The impulse remains active enough to produce another impulse during myocardial repolarization.	♥ Coronary artery disease ♥ Cardiomyopathy ♥ Myocardial infarction
Afterdepolarization	♥ An injured cell only partly repolarizes. ♥ Partial repolarization can lead to a repetitive ectopic firing called *triggered activity*. ♥ Triggered activity produces depolarization and can lead to atrial or ventricular tachycardia.	♥ Cell injury ♥ Digoxin toxicity

Spark plugs, belts, and fluids look fine. Must be a timing problem.

Premature atrial contractions

PACs originate from an irritable spot, or *focus*, in the atria that takes over as pacemaker for one or more beats. In a patient with heart disease, PACs may lead to more serious arrhythmias, such as atrial fibrillation and atrial flutter. In a patient who has had an acute MI, PACs can serve as an early sign of heart failure or an electrolyte imbalance.

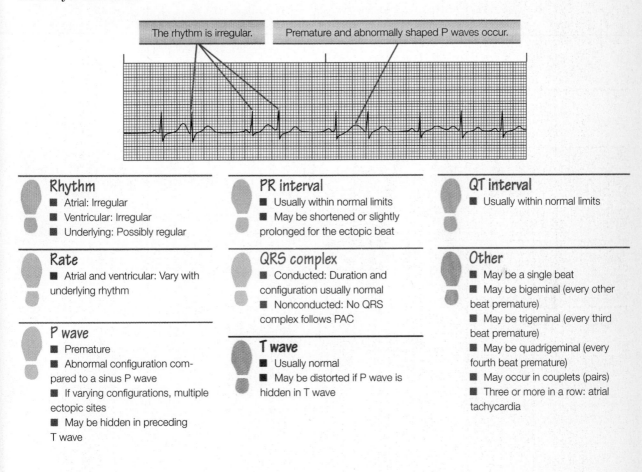

The rhythm is irregular.

Premature and abnormally shaped P waves occur.

Rhythm
- Atrial: Irregular
- Ventricular: Irregular
- Underlying: Possibly regular

Rate
- Atrial and ventricular: Vary with underlying rhythm

P wave
- Premature
- Abnormal configuration compared to a sinus P wave
- If varying configurations, multiple ectopic sites
- May be hidden in preceding T wave

PR interval
- Usually within normal limits
- May be shortened or slightly prolonged for the ectopic beat

QRS complex
- Conducted: Duration and configuration usually normal
- Nonconducted: No QRS complex follows PAC

T wave
- Usually normal
- May be distorted if P wave is hidden in T wave

QT interval
- Usually within normal limits

Other
- May be a single beat
- May be bigeminal (every other beat premature)
- May be trigeminal (every third beat premature)
- May be quadrigeminal (every fourth beat premature)
- May occur in couplets (pairs)
- Three or more in a row: atrial tachycardia

Atrial tachycardia

Atrial tachycardia is a supraventricular tachycardia characterized by an atrial rate of 150 to 250 beats/minute. Three types of atrial tachycardia exist: atrial tachycardia with block, multifocal atrial tachycardia (MAT, or *chaotic atrial rhythm*), and paroxysmal atrial tachycardia (PAT). In atrial tachycardia with block, the number of P waves for each QRS complex may vary, depending if the block is regular. The most common block is a 2:1, with two atrial contractions for every ventricular contraction. In MAT, the P waves vary and atrial and ventricular contractions are irregular. The distinguishing characteristic of PAT is that tachycardia starts and stops suddenly in periods of normal sinus rhythm.

The P wave may hide in the preceding T wave.

The rate is between 150 and 250 beats/minute.

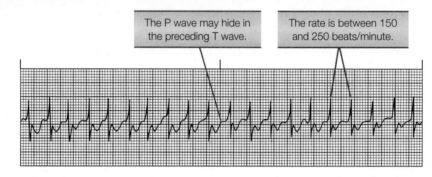

 ### Rhythm
■ Atrial: Usually regular
■ Ventricular: Regular or irregular depending on AV conduction ratio and type of atrial tachycardia

Rate
■ Atrial: Three or more consecutive ectopic atrial beats at 150 to 250 beats/minute; rarely exceeds 250 beats/minute
■ Ventricular: Varies, depending on AV conduction ratio

P wave
■ Deviates from normal appearance
■ May be hidden in preceding T wave
■ If visible, usually upright and precedes each QRS complex

 ### PR interval
■ May be difficult to measure if P wave can't be distinguished from preceding T wave

QRS complex
■ Usually normal duration and configuration
■ May be abnormal if impulses conducted abnormally through ventricles

T wave
■ Usually visible
■ May be distorted by P wave
■ May be inverted if ischemia is present

QT interval
■ Usually within normal limits
■ May be shorter because of rapid rate

Other
■ May be difficult to differentiate atrial tachycardia with block from sinus arrhythmia with U waves

Atrial flutter

Atrial flutter, a supraventricular tachycardia, is characterized by an atrial rate of 250 to 400 beats/minute, although it's generally around 300 beats/minute. The clinical significance of atrial flutter is determined by the number of impulses conducted through the node — expressed as a conduction ratio (for example, 2:1 or 4:1) — and the resulting ventricular rate. If the ventricular rate is too slow (less than 40 beats/minute) or too fast (more than 150 beats/minute), cardiac output can be seriously compromised. Usually, the faster the ventricular rate, the more dangerous the arrhythmia.

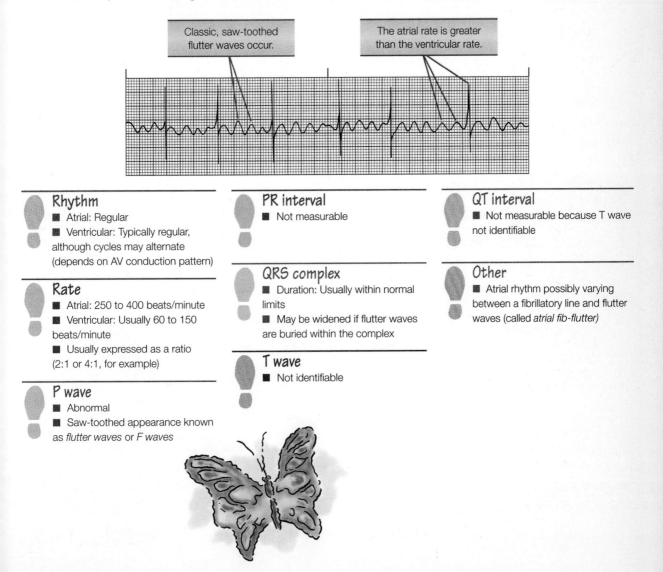

Classic, saw-toothed flutter waves occur.

The atrial rate is greater than the ventricular rate.

Rhythm
- Atrial: Regular
- Ventricular: Typically regular, although cycles may alternate (depends on AV conduction pattern)

Rate
- Atrial: 250 to 400 beats/minute
- Ventricular: Usually 60 to 150 beats/minute
- Usually expressed as a ratio (2:1 or 4:1, for example)

P wave
- Abnormal
- Saw-toothed appearance known as *flutter waves* or *F waves*

PR interval
- Not measurable

QRS complex
- Duration: Usually within normal limits
- May be widened if flutter waves are buried within the complex

T wave
- Not identifiable

QT interval
- Not measurable because T wave not identifiable

Other
- Atrial rhythm possibly varying between a fibrillatory line and flutter waves (called *atrial fib-flutter*)

Atrial fibrillation

Sometimes called *A-fib*, atrial fibrillation is defined as chaotic, asynchronous electrical activity in the atrial tissue. This rhythm may be sustained or paroxysmal (occurring in bursts). Atrial fibrillation eliminates atrial kick. If the ventricular response is greater than 100 beats/minute — a condition called *uncontrolled atrial fibrillation* — the patient may develop heart failure, angina, or syncope. A patient with preexisting cardiac disease may develop shock and severe heart failure.

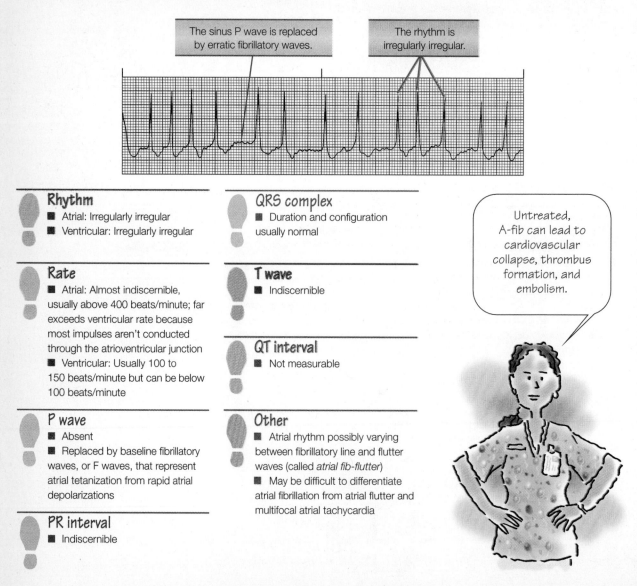

The sinus P wave is replaced by erratic fibrillatory waves.

The rhythm is irregularly irregular.

Untreated, A-fib can lead to cardiovascular collapse, thrombus formation, and embolism.

Rhythm
- Atrial: Irregularly irregular
- Ventricular: Irregularly irregular

Rate
- Atrial: Almost indiscernible, usually above 400 beats/minute; far exceeds ventricular rate because most impulses aren't conducted through the atrioventricular junction
- Ventricular: Usually 100 to 150 beats/minute but can be below 100 beats/minute

P wave
- Absent
- Replaced by baseline fibrillatory waves, or F waves, that represent atrial tetanization from rapid atrial depolarizations

PR interval
- Indiscernible

QRS complex
- Duration and configuration usually normal

T wave
- Indiscernible

QT interval
- Not measurable

Other
- Atrial rhythm possibly varying between fibrillatory line and flutter waves (called *atrial fib-flutter*)
- May be difficult to differentiate atrial fibrillation from atrial flutter and multifocal atrial tachycardia

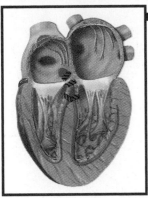

AV block

The severity, or degree, of an AV block is measured according to how well the node conducts impulses.

AV heart block results from an interruption in the conduction of impulses between the atria and ventricles. It can be total or partial; can delay conduction; and can occur at the AV node, bundle of His, or bundle branches. When impulses from the SA node are blocked at the AV node or below, atrial rates are commonly normal (60 to 100 beats/minute). The clinical effects of the block depend on how many impulses are completely blocked, how slow the resulting ventricular rate is, and how the block ultimately affects the heart. A slow ventricular rate can decrease cardiac output, possibly causing light-headedness, hypotension, and confusion.

Comparing degrees of AV block

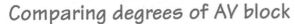

Type	Distinguishing characteristic	Possible causes
First	♥PR interval > 0.20 second	♥Degenerative changes ♥Drugs: beta-adrenergic blockers, calcium channel blockers, digoxin ♥MI ♥Myocarditis
Type I second-degree	♥Progressive prolongation of PR interval until P wave occurs without a QRS complex (dropped beat)	♥CAD ♥Drugs: beta-adrenergic blockers, calcium channel blockers, digoxin ♥Increased parasympathetic tone ♥Inferior-wall MI ♥Rheumatic fever
Type II second-degree	♥Constant PR interval for conducted beats ♥Periodic nonconducted P wave (dropped beat)	♥Anterior-wall MI ♥Degenerative changes in conduction system ♥Organic heart disease ♥Severe CAD
Third degree	♥No relationship between P wave and QRS complex ♥Independent beating of atria and ventricles	**At AV node level** ♥AV node damage ♥Increased parasympathetic tone ♥Inferior-wall MI ♥Drug toxicity **At infranodal level** ♥Extensive anterior-wall MI

First-degree AV block

First-degree AV block occurs when impulses from the atria are consistently delayed during conduction through the AV node. The least dangerous type of AV block, first-degree AV block can progress to a more severe block.

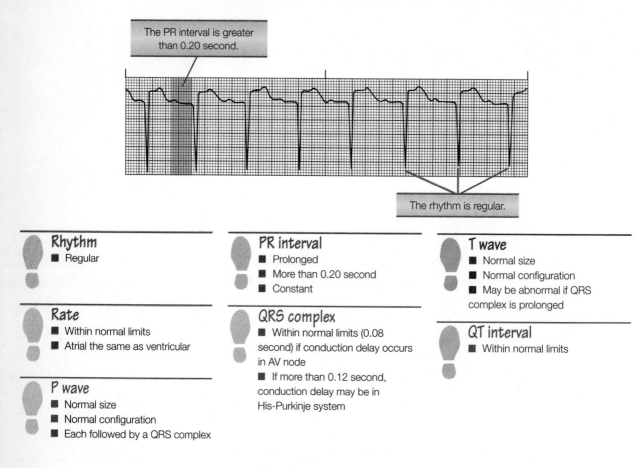

The PR interval is greater than 0.20 second.

The rhythm is regular.

Rhythm
■ Regular

Rate
■ Within normal limits
■ Atrial the same as ventricular

P wave
■ Normal size
■ Normal configuration
■ Each followed by a QRS complex

PR interval
■ Prolonged
■ More than 0.20 second
■ Constant

QRS complex
■ Within normal limits (0.08 second) if conduction delay occurs in AV node
■ If more than 0.12 second, conduction delay may be in His-Purkinje system

T wave
■ Normal size
■ Normal configuration
■ May be abnormal if QRS complex is prolonged

QT interval
■ Within normal limits

Type I second-degree AV block

Also called *Wenckebach* or *Mobitz type I block*, type I second-degree AV block occurs when each successive impulse from the SA node is delayed slightly longer than the previous impulse. That pattern continues until an impulse fails to be conducted to the ventricles, and the cycle then repeats.

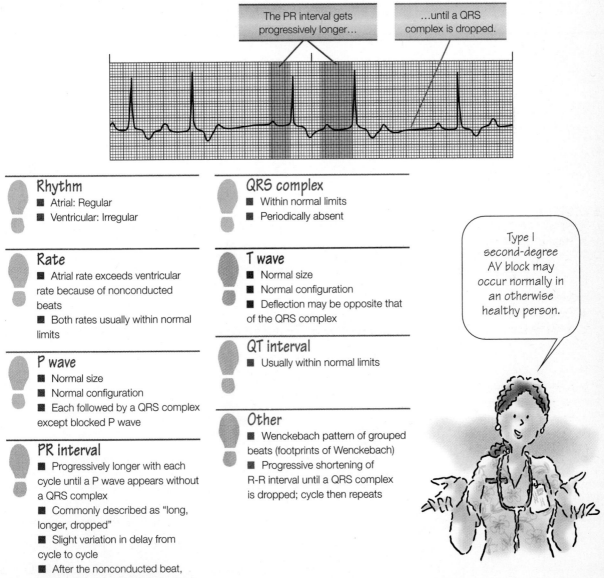

The PR interval gets progressively longer…

…until a QRS complex is dropped.

Rhythm
- Atrial: Regular
- Ventricular: Irregular

Rate
- Atrial rate exceeds ventricular rate because of nonconducted beats
- Both rates usually within normal limits

P wave
- Normal size
- Normal configuration
- Each followed by a QRS complex except blocked P wave

PR interval
- Progressively longer with each cycle until a P wave appears without a QRS complex
- Commonly described as "long, longer, dropped"
- Slight variation in delay from cycle to cycle
- After the nonconducted beat, shorter than the interval preceding it

QRS complex
- Within normal limits
- Periodically absent

T wave
- Normal size
- Normal configuration
- Deflection may be opposite that of the QRS complex

QT interval
- Usually within normal limits

Other
- Wenckebach pattern of grouped beats (footprints of Wenckebach)
- Progressive shortening of R-R interval until a QRS complex is dropped; cycle then repeats

Type I second-degree AV block may occur normally in an otherwise healthy person.

Type II second-degree AV block

Type II second-degree AV block, also known as *Mobitz type II block*, is less common than type I but is more serious. The ventricular rate tends to be slower than in type I and cardiac output is diminished. It's also more likely to cause symptoms and progress to a more serious form of block.

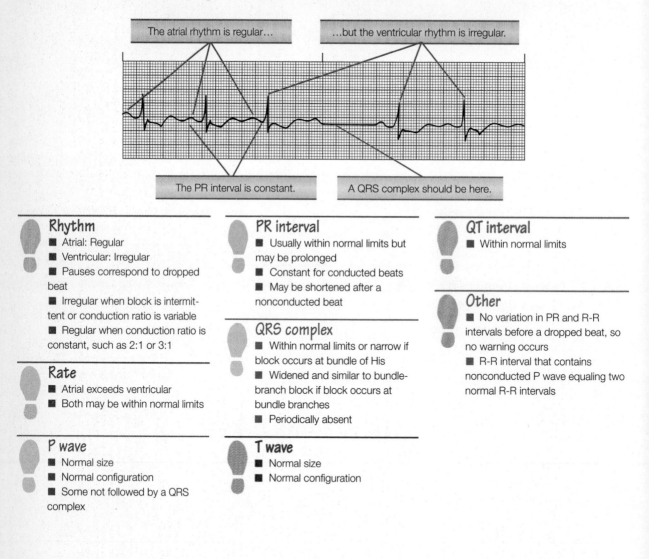

The atrial rhythm is regular...

...but the ventricular rhythm is irregular.

The PR interval is constant.

A QRS complex should be here.

Rhythm
- Atrial: Regular
- Ventricular: Irregular
- Pauses correspond to dropped beat
- Irregular when block is intermittent or conduction ratio is variable
- Regular when conduction ratio is constant, such as 2:1 or 3:1

Rate
- Atrial exceeds ventricular
- Both may be within normal limits

P wave
- Normal size
- Normal configuration
- Some not followed by a QRS complex

PR interval
- Usually within normal limits but may be prolonged
- Constant for conducted beats
- May be shortened after a nonconducted beat

QRS complex
- Within normal limits or narrow if block occurs at bundle of His
- Widened and similar to bundle-branch block if block occurs at bundle branches
- Periodically absent

T wave
- Normal size
- Normal configuration

QT interval
- Within normal limits

Other
- No variation in PR and R-R intervals before a dropped beat, so no warning occurs
- R-R interval that contains nonconducted P wave equaling two normal R-R intervals

Third-degree AV block

Also called *complete heart block*, third-degree AV block occurs when impulses from the atria are completely blocked at the AV node and can't be conducted to the ventricles. The ventricular rhythm may originate from the AV node or the Purkinje system. Diminished cardiac output may cause poor exercise tolerance and shortness of breath in patients with very slow ventricular rates. More serious symptoms, including syncope, chest pain, and hypotension, are also common.

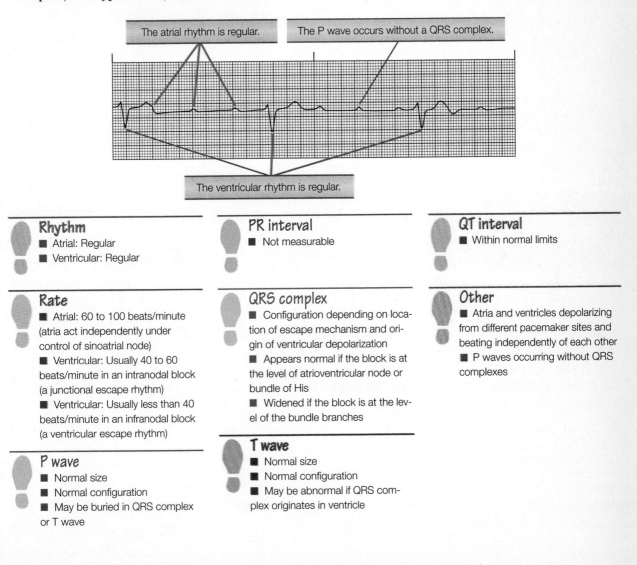

The atrial rhythm is regular.

The P wave occurs without a QRS complex.

The ventricular rhythm is regular.

Rhythm
- Atrial: Regular
- Ventricular: Regular

Rate
- Atrial: 60 to 100 beats/minute (atria act independently under control of sinoatrial node)
- Ventricular: Usually 40 to 60 beats/minute in an intranodal block (a junctional escape rhythm)
- Ventricular: Usually less than 40 beats/minute in an infranodal block (a ventricular escape rhythm)

P wave
- Normal size
- Normal configuration
- May be buried in QRS complex or T wave

PR interval
- Not measurable

QRS complex
- Configuration depending on location of escape mechanism and origin of ventricular depolarization
- Appears normal if the block is at the level of atrioventricular node or bundle of His
- Widened if the block is at the level of the bundle branches

T wave
- Normal size
- Normal configuration
- May be abnormal if QRS complex originates in ventricle

QT interval
- Within normal limits

Other
- Atria and ventricles depolarizing from different pacemaker sites and beating independently of each other
- P waves occurring without QRS complexes

Hey wait! I thought retro was in!

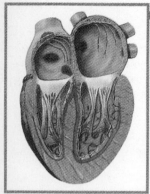

Junctional arrhythmias

Junctional arrhythmias originate in the AV junction—the area around the AV node and the bundle of His. These arrhythmias occur when the SA node fails to conduct impulses or when a block in conduction occurs. Electrical impulses may then be initiated by pacemaker cells in the AV junction in the middle of the heart. Impulses generated in this area cause the heart to depolarize abnormally. The impulse moves upward and causes backward, or retrograde, depolarization of the atria, resulting in inverted (rather than upright) P waves in leads II, III, and aV_F. The ventricles respond normally to the stimulus, resulting in a QRS complex that appears normal on the rhythm strip.

P wave positions

The position of the P wave depends on whether the impulse reaches the atria or ventricles first.

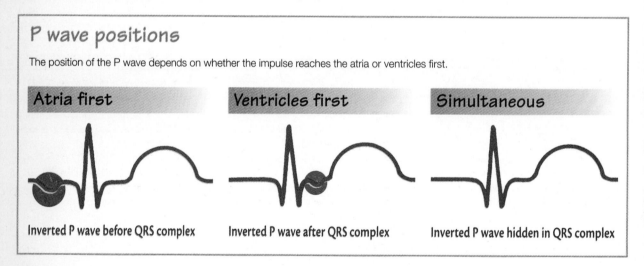

Atria first	Ventricles first	Simultaneous
Inverted P wave before QRS complex	Inverted P wave after QRS complex	Inverted P wave hidden in QRS complex

Premature junctional contractions

A PJC is a beat that occurs before a normal sinus beat and causes an irregular rhythm. This ectopic beat occurs when an irritable location within the AV junction acts as a pacemaker and fires either prematurely or out of sequence. Although the junctional beat itself isn't recorded on the ECG strip, its effects on the timing of atrial (retrograde) and ventricular (anterograde) depolarization are seen.

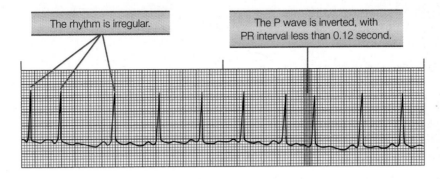

The rhythm is irregular.

The P wave is inverted, with PR interval less than 0.12 second.

Rhythm
- Atrial: Irregular during PJCs
- Ventricular: Irregular during PJCs
- Underlying rhythm possibly regular

Rate
- Atrial: Reflects underlying rhythm
- Ventricular: Reflects underlying rhythm

P wave
- Usually inverted (leads II, III, and aV$_F$)
- May occur before, during, or after QRS complex, depending on initial direction of depolarization
- May be hidden in QRS complex

PR interval
- Shortened (less than 0.12 second) if P wave precedes QRS complex
- Not measurable if no P wave precedes QRS complex

QRS complex
- Usually normal configuration and duration because ventricles usually depolarize normally

T wave
- Usually normal configuration

QT interval
- Usually within normal limits

Other
- Commonly accompanied by a compensatory pause, reflecting retrograde atrial conduction

Junctional escape rhythm

A junctional escape rhythm is a string of beats that occurs after a conduction delay from the atria. It can be caused by any condition that disturbs SA node function or enhances AV junction automaticity. A patient with a junctional escape rhythm has a slow, regular pulse rate of 40 to 60 beats/minute and may be asymptomatic.

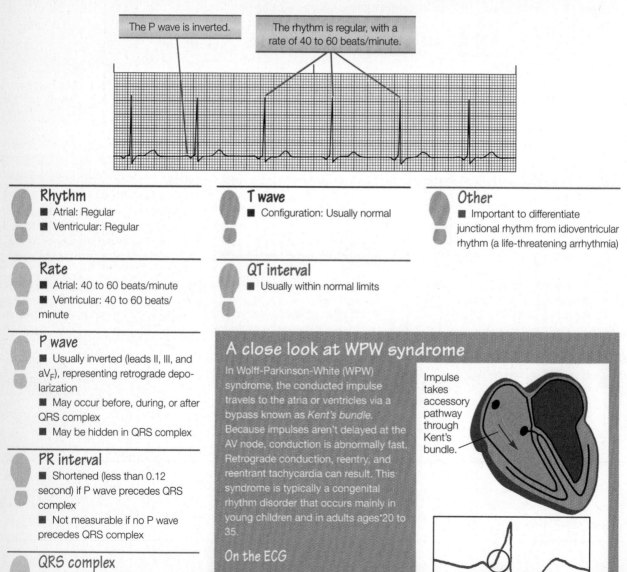

The P wave is inverted.

The rhythm is regular, with a rate of 40 to 60 beats/minute.

Rhythm
- Atrial: Regular
- Ventricular: Regular

Rate
- Atrial: 40 to 60 beats/minute
- Ventricular: 40 to 60 beats/minute

P wave
- Usually inverted (leads II, III, and aV$_F$), representing retrograde depolarization
- May occur before, during, or after QRS complex
- May be hidden in QRS complex

PR interval
- Shortened (less than 0.12 second) if P wave precedes QRS complex
- Not measurable if no P wave precedes QRS complex

QRS complex
- Duration: Usually within normal limits
- Configuration: Usually normal

T wave
- Configuration: Usually normal

QT interval
- Usually within normal limits

Other
- Important to differentiate junctional rhythm from idioventricular rhythm (a life-threatening arrhythmia)

A close look at WPW syndrome

In Wolff-Parkinson-White (WPW) syndrome, the conducted impulse travels to the atria or ventricles via a bypass known as *Kent's bundle*. Because impulses aren't delayed at the AV node, conduction is abnormally fast. Retrograde conduction, reentry, and reentrant tachycardia can result. This syndrome is typically a congenital rhythm disorder that occurs mainly in young children and in adults ages 20 to 35.

On the ECG
- Delta wave (hallmark sign)
- Short PR interval (< 0.10 second)
- Wide QRS complex (> 0.10 second)

Impulse takes accessory pathway through Kent's bundle.

Delta wave

Accelerated junctional rhythm

An accelerated junctional rhythm results when an irritable focus in the AV junction speeds up and takes over as the heart's pacemaker. The atria depolarize by retrograde conduction, and the ventricles depolarize normally. The accelerated rate is usually 60 to 100 beats/minute.

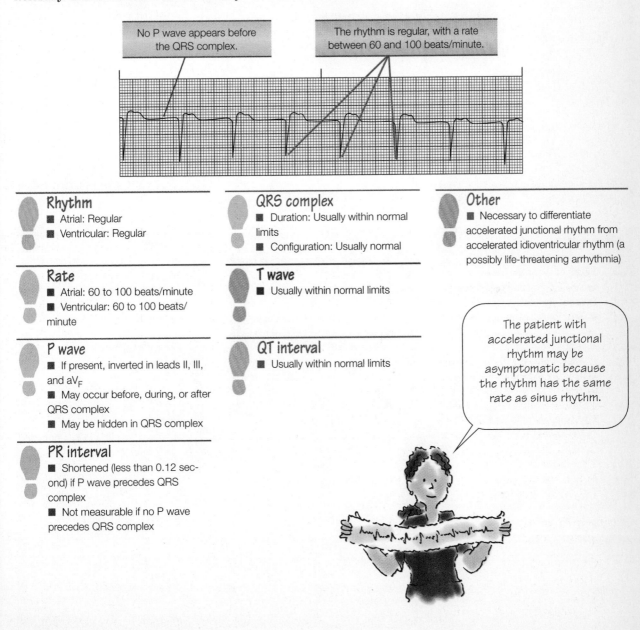

No P wave appears before the QRS complex.

The rhythm is regular, with a rate between 60 and 100 beats/minute.

Rhythm
- Atrial: Regular
- Ventricular: Regular

Rate
- Atrial: 60 to 100 beats/minute
- Ventricular: 60 to 100 beats/minute

P wave
- If present, inverted in leads II, III, and aV$_F$
- May occur before, during, or after QRS complex
- May be hidden in QRS complex

PR interval
- Shortened (less than 0.12 second) if P wave precedes QRS complex
- Not measurable if no P wave precedes QRS complex

QRS complex
- Duration: Usually within normal limits
- Configuration: Usually normal

T wave
- Usually within normal limits

QT interval
- Usually within normal limits

Other
- Necessary to differentiate accelerated junctional rhythm from accelerated idioventricular rhythm (a possibly life-threatening arrhythmia)

The patient with accelerated junctional rhythm may be asymptomatic because the rhythm has the same rate as sinus rhythm.

Junctional tachycardia

In junctional tachycardia, three or more PJCs occur in a row. This supraventricular tachycardia occurs when an irritable focus from the AV junction overrides the SA node's ability to function as the heart's pacemaker. The atria depolarize by retrograde conduction; however, conduction through the ventricles remains normal.

The rhythm is regular, with a rate of 100 to 200 beats/minute.

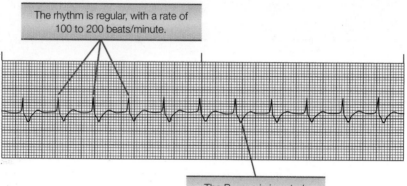

The P wave is inverted.

Rhythm
- Atrial: Usually regular but may be difficult to determine if P wave is hidden in QRS complex or preceding T wave
- Ventricular: Usually regular

Rate
- Atrial: Exceeds 100 beats/minute (usually 100 to 200 beats/minute) but may be difficult to determine if P wave isn't visible
- Ventricular: Exceeds 100 beats/minute (usually 100 to 200 beats/minute)

P wave
- Usually inverted in leads II, III, and aV$_F$
- May occur before, during, or after QRS complex
- May be hidden in QRS complex

PR interval
- Shortened (less than 0.12 second) if P wave precedes QRS complex
- Not measurable if no P wave precedes QRS complex

QRS complex
- Duration: Within normal limits
- Configuration: Usually normal

T wave
- Configuration: Usually normal
- May be abnormal if P wave is hidden in T wave
- May be indiscernible because of fast rate

QT interval
- Usually within normal limits

Other
- Onset possibly gradual (nonparoxysmal) or sudden (paroxysmal)

Bundle-branch block

In bundle-branch block (BBB), the left or the right bundle branch fails to conduct impulses. A BBB that occurs low in the left bundle is called a *hemiblock* or *fascicular block.* In BBB, the impulse travels down the unaffected bundle branch and then from one myocardial cell to the next to depolarize the ventricle. Because this cell-to-cell conduction progresses much slower than the conduction along the specialized cells of the conduction system, ventricular depolarization is prolonged.

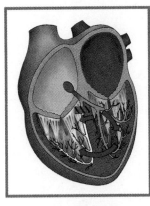

Right bundle-branch block

Right bundle-branch block (RBBB) may occur in patients with CAD, pulmonary embolism, or recent anterior-wall MI. However, it can also occur without the presence of cardiac disease.

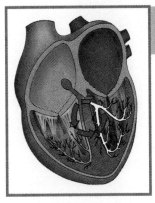

Left bundle-branch block

Left bundle-branch block (LBBB) never occurs normally. This block is usually caused by hypertensive heart disease, aortic stenosis, degenerative changes of the conduction system, or CAD.

Recognizing RBBB and LBBB

The normal width of a QRS complex is 0.06 to 0.10 second. However, prolonged ventricular depolarization widens the QRS complex. If the width increases to greater than 0.12 second, a bundle-branch block is present.

After you identify a BBB, examine lead V_1, which lies to the right of the heart, and lead V_6, which lies to the left of the heart. You'll use these leads to determine whether the block is a right bundle-branch block (RBBB) or a left bundle-branch block (LBBB).

RBBB

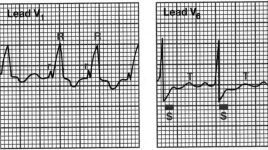

In RBBB, V_1 shows a small r wave (showing left ventricular depolarization), followed by a large R wave (confirming right ventricular depolarization). V_6 shows a widened S wave and an upright T wave.

LBBB

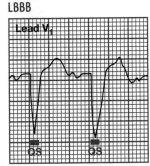
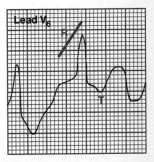

In LBBB, V_1 shows no R wave and a wide, large QS wave. V_6 shows slurred R waves and inverted T waves.

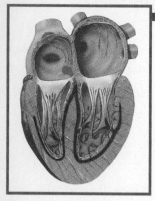

Ventricular arrhythmias

Ventricular arrhythmias originate in the ventricles below the bundle of His. They occur when electrical impulses depolarize the myocardium using an abnormal pathway. When electrical impulses originate in the ventricles instead of the atria, atrial kick is lost and cardiac output decreases by as much as 30%. As a result, patients may show signs and symptoms of cardiac decompensation, including hypotension, angina, syncope, and respiratory distress.

Ventricular arrhythmias are potentially deadly because the ventricles are ultimately responsible for cardiac output. Rapid recognition and treatment of ventricular arrhythmias increase the chance for successful resuscitation.

Signs and symptoms of cardiac decompensation

Hypotension and syncope

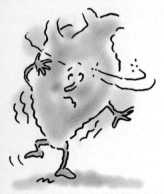

Respiratory distress

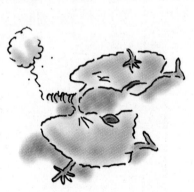

Angina

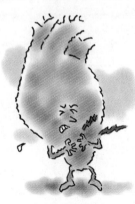

Premature ventricular contractions

A PVC is an ectopic beat that originates low in the ventricles and occurs earlier than normal. PVCs can occur singly, in clusters of two or more, or in repeating patterns, such as bigeminy or trigeminy. PVCs that look alike are called *unifocal* and originate from the same ectopic focus. These beats may appear in patterns that can progress to more lethal arrhythmias.

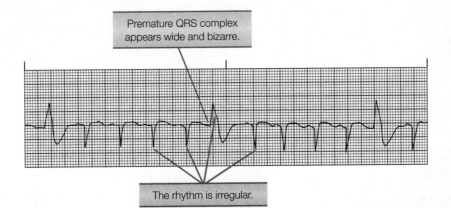

Premature QRS complex appears wide and bizarre.

The rhythm is irregular.

Rhythm
- Atrial: Irregular during PVCs
- Ventricular: Irregular during PVCs
- Underlying rhythm may be regular

Rate
- Atrial: Reflects underlying rhythm
- Ventricular: Reflects underlying rhythm

P wave
- Usually absent in ectopic beat
- May appear after QRS complex with retrograde conduction to atria
- Usually normal if present in underlying rhythm

PR interval
- Not measurable except in underlying rhythm

QRS complex
- Occurs earlier than expected
- Duration: Exceeds 0.12 second
- Configuration: Bizarre and wide but usually normal in underlying rhythm

T wave
- Opposite direction to QRS complex
- May trigger more serious rhythm disturbances when PVC occurs on the downslope of the preceding normal T wave (R-on-T phenomenon)

QT interval
- Not usually measured except in underlying rhythm

Other
- PVC possibly followed by full or incomplete compensatory pause
- Interpolated PVC: Occurring between two normally conducted QRS complexes without great disturbance to underlying rhythm
- Full compensatory pause absent with interpolated PVCs

Patterns of potentially dangerous PVCs

Paired PVCs

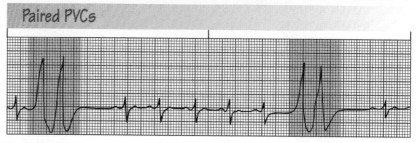

Two PVCs in a row, called *paired PVCs* or a *ventricular couplet*, can produce VT because the second contraction usually meets refractory tissue. A burst, or *salvo*, of three or more PVCs in a row is considered a run of VT.

Multiform PVCs

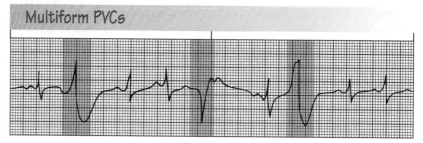

Multiform PVCs look different from one another and arise either from different sites or from the same site via abnormal conduction. Multiform PVCs may indicate severe heart disease or digoxin toxicity.

Bigeminy and trigeminy

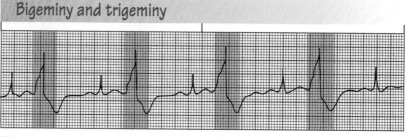

PVCs that occur every other beat (bigeminy) or every third beat (trigeminy) can result in VT or VF.

R-on-T phenomenon

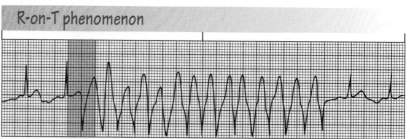

In R-on-T phenomenon, a PVC occurs so early that it falls on the T wave of the preceding beat. Because the cells haven't fully repolarized, VT or VF can result.

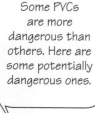

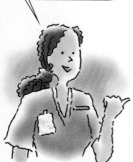

Some PVCs are more dangerous than others. Here are some potentially dangerous ones.

Take this info to heart

♥ Until effective treatment begins, patients with PVCs accompanied by serious symptoms should have continuous ECG monitoring and ambulate only with assistance.

♥ If the patient is discharged from the hospital on antiarrhythmic medications, make sure family members know how to contact the emergency medical system and perform cardiopulmonary resuscitation.

Ventricular tachycardia

In VT, commonly called *V-tach*, three or more PVCs occur in a row. This arrhythmia usually precedes ventricular fibrillation and sudden cardiac death, especially in patients who aren't in the hospital. It can occur in short, paroxysmal bursts lasting fewer than 30 seconds and causing few or no symptoms. Alternatively, it can be sustained, requiring immediate treatment to prevent death.

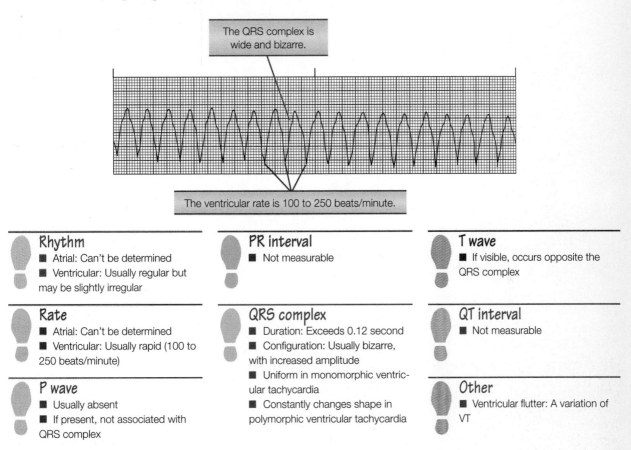

The QRS complex is wide and bizarre.

The ventricular rate is 100 to 250 beats/minute.

Rhythm
- Atrial: Can't be determined
- Ventricular: Usually regular but may be slightly irregular

Rate
- Atrial: Can't be determined
- Ventricular: Usually rapid (100 to 250 beats/minute)

P wave
- Usually absent
- If present, not associated with QRS complex

PR interval
- Not measurable

QRS complex
- Duration: Exceeds 0.12 second
- Configuration: Usually bizarre, with increased amplitude
- Uniform in monomorphic ventricular tachycardia
- Constantly changes shape in polymorphic ventricular tachycardia

T wave
- If visible, occurs opposite the QRS complex

QT interval
- Not measurable

Other
- Ventricular flutter: A variation of VT

Torsades de pointes

Torsades de pointes is a special variation of polymorphic VT that may deteriorate into VF. The cause is usually reversible—most commonly, use of drugs that lengthen the QT interval, such as quinidine, procainamide, and sotalol (Betapace). Myocardial ischemia and electrolyte imbalances can also cause this arrhythmia.

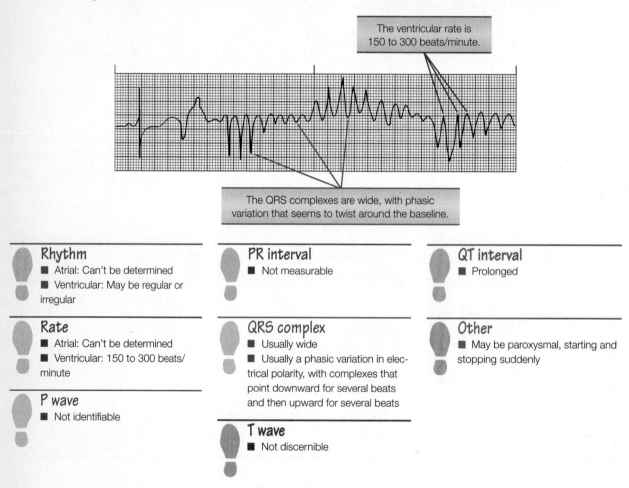

The ventricular rate is 150 to 300 beats/minute.

The QRS complexes are wide, with phasic variation that seems to twist around the baseline.

Rhythm
- Atrial: Can't be determined
- Ventricular: May be regular or irregular

Rate
- Atrial: Can't be determined
- Ventricular: 150 to 300 beats/minute

P wave
- Not identifiable

PR interval
- Not measurable

QRS complex
- Usually wide
- Usually a phasic variation in electrical polarity, with complexes that point downward for several beats and then upward for several beats

T wave
- Not discernible

QT interval
- Prolonged

Other
- May be paroxysmal, starting and stopping suddenly

Ventricular fibrillation

VF, commonly called *V-fib*, is a chaotic pattern of electrical activity in the ventricles in which electrical impulses arise from many different foci. The ventricles quiver instead of contracting, so cardiac output falls to zero. If fibrillation continues, it leads to ventricular standstill and death.

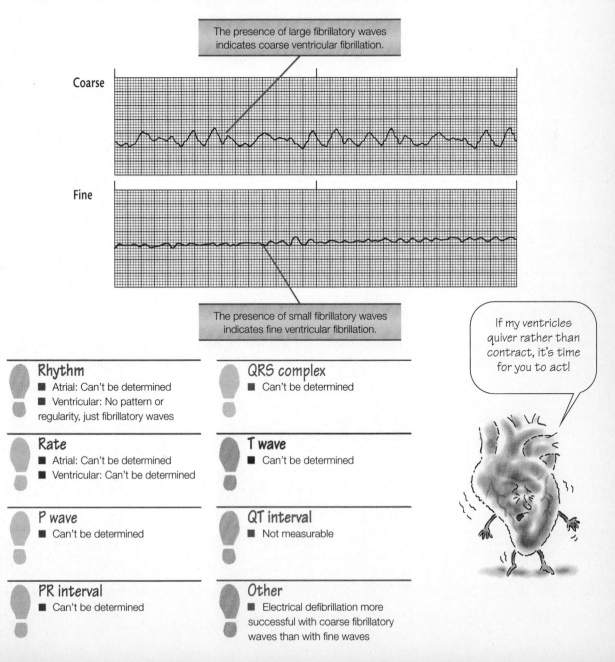

The presence of large fibrillatory waves indicates coarse ventricular fibrillation.

Coarse

Fine

The presence of small fibrillatory waves indicates fine ventricular fibrillation.

If my ventricles quiver rather than contract, it's time for you to act!

Rhythm
■ Atrial: Can't be determined
■ Ventricular: No pattern or regularity, just fibrillatory waves

Rate
■ Atrial: Can't be determined
■ Ventricular: Can't be determined

P wave
■ Can't be determined

PR interval
■ Can't be determined

QRS complex
■ Can't be determined

T wave
■ Can't be determined

QT interval
■ Not measurable

Other
■ Electrical defibrillation more successful with coarse fibrillatory waves than with fine waves

Idioventricular arrhythmia

Called the *rhythm of last resort,* idioventricular arrhythmia acts as safety mechanisms to prevent ventricular standstill when no impulses are conducted to the ventricles from above the bundle of His. The cells of the His-Purkinje system take over and act as the heart's pacemaker to generate electrical impulses.

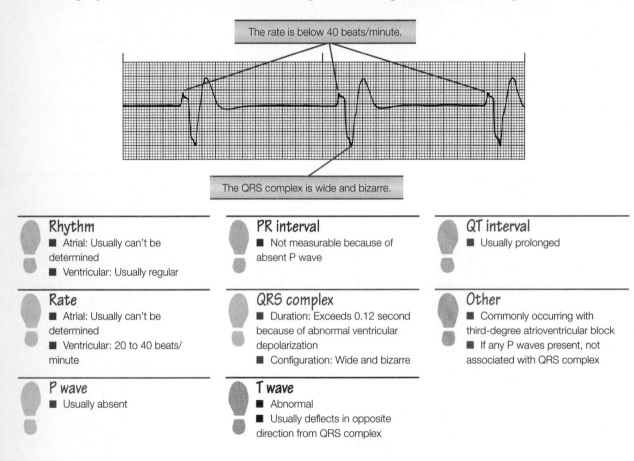

The rate is below 40 beats/minute.

The QRS complex is wide and bizarre.

Rhythm
■ Atrial: Usually can't be determined
■ Ventricular: Usually regular

Rate
■ Atrial: Usually can't be determined
■ Ventricular: 20 to 40 beats/minute

P wave
■ Usually absent

PR interval
■ Not measurable because of absent P wave

QRS complex
■ Duration: Exceeds 0.12 second because of abnormal ventricular depolarization
■ Configuration: Wide and bizarre

T wave
■ Abnormal
■ Usually deflects in opposite direction from QRS complex

QT interval
■ Usually prolonged

Other
■ Commonly occurring with third-degree atrioventricular block
■ If any P waves present, not associated with QRS complex

Asystole

Asystole is ventricular standstill. The patient is completely unresponsive, with no electrical activity in the heart, no cardiac output, and no respirations.

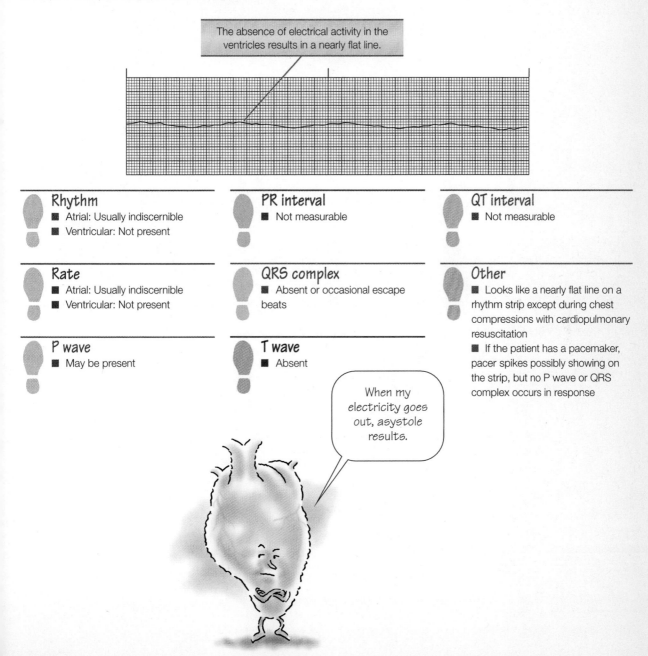

The absence of electrical activity in the ventricles results in a nearly flat line.

Rhythm
- Atrial: Usually indiscernible
- Ventricular: Not present

Rate
- Atrial: Usually indiscernible
- Ventricular: Not present

P wave
- May be present

PR interval
- Not measurable

QRS complex
- Absent or occasional escape beats

T wave
- Absent

QT interval
- Not measurable

Other
- Looks like a nearly flat line on a rhythm strip except during chest compressions with cardiopulmonary resuscitation
- If the patient has a pacemaker, pacer spikes possibly showing on the strip, but no P wave or QRS complex occurs in response

When my electricity goes out, asystole results.

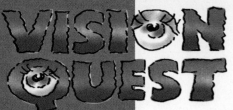

Color my world

Color each circle with the appropriate lead color that should be used for continuous cardiac monitoring.

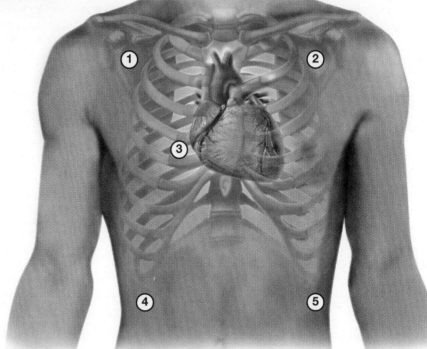

Matchmaker

Match each of the arrhythmias shown with their correct name.

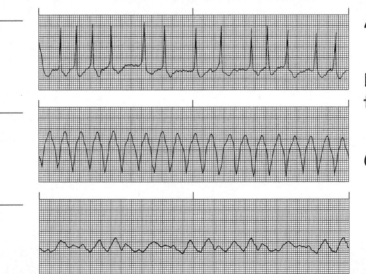

1. _____   **A.** VF

2. _____   **B.** Atrial fibrillation

3. _____   **C.** VT

Answers: Color my world 1. White, 2. Black, 3. Brown, 4. Green, 5. Red
Matchmaker 1. B, 2. C, 3. A.

5 Hemodynamic monitoring

A star must always remember to wave to her fans.

Arterial blood pressure monitoring

Hemodynamic monitoring is used to assess cardiac function and determine the effectiveness of therapy. In arterial blood pressure monitoring, a doctor inserts a catheter into the patient's radial or femoral artery to measure systolic, diastolic, and mean pressures or to

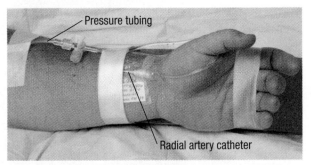

Pressure tubing

Radial artery catheter

obtain samples for ABG studies. A transducer transforms the flow of blood during systole and diastole into a waveform, which appears on a monitor screen.

Normal arterial pressure parameters

In general, arterial systolic pressure reflects the peak pressure generated by the left ventricle. It also indicates compliance of the large arteries, or the *peripheral resistance.*

Arterial diastolic pressure reflects the runoff velocity and elasticity of the arterial system, particularly the arterioles.

Mean arterial pressure (MAP) is the average pressure in the arterial system during systole and diastole. It reflects the driving, or *perfusion,* pressure and is determined by arterial blood volume and blood vessel elasticity and resistance.

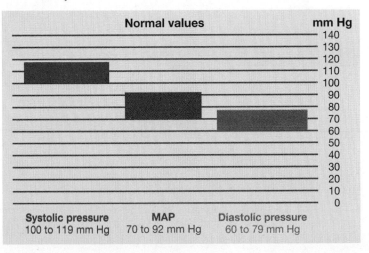

Normal values   **mm Hg**

	140
	130
	120
	110
	100
	90
	80
	70
	60
	50
	40
	30
	20
	10
	0

Systolic pressure **MAP** **Diastolic pressure**
100 to 119 mm Hg 70 to 92 mm Hg 60 to 79 mm Hg

$$MAP = \frac{\text{systolic pressure} + 2\,(\text{diastolic pressure})}{3}$$

Arterial waveform configuration

Normal arterial blood pressure produces a characteristic waveform, representing ventricular systole and diastole. The waveform has five distinct components, as shown below.

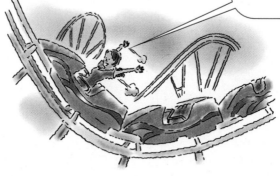

Knowing the components of an arterial waveform keeps you ahead of the game on arterial pressure monitoring.

Normal arterial waveform

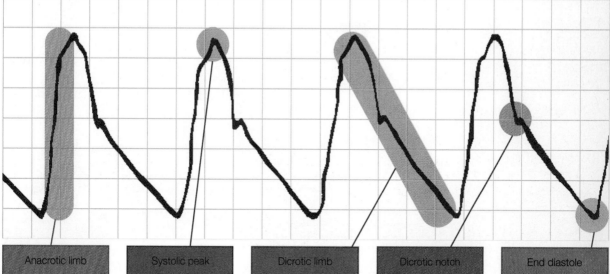

Anacrotic limb	Systolic peak	Dicrotic limb	Dicrotic notch	End diastole
The *anacrotic limb* marks the waveform's initial upstroke, which occurs as blood is rapidly ejected from the ventricle through the open aortic valve into the aorta.	Arterial pressure then rises sharply, resulting in the *systolic peak*—the waveform's highest point.	As blood continues into the peripheral vessels, arterial pressure falls and the waveform begins a downward trend, called the *dicrotic limb*. Arterial pressure usually keeps falling until pressure in the ventricle is less than pressure in the aortic root.	When ventricular pressure is lower than aortic root pressure, the aortic valve closes. This event appears as a small notch on the waveform's downside, called the *dicrotic notch*.	When the aortic valve closes, diastole begins, progressing until aortic root pressure gradually falls to its lowest point. On the waveform, this is known as *end diastole*.

Recognizing abnormal waveforms

Understanding a normal arterial waveform is relatively straightforward. Unfortunately, an abnormal waveform isn't so easy to decipher. Abnormal patterns and markings, however, may provide important diagnostic clues to the patient's cardiovascular status, or they may simply signal trouble in the monitor. Use this chart to help you recognize waveform abnormalities. Always check the patient when an abnormal waveform is noted.

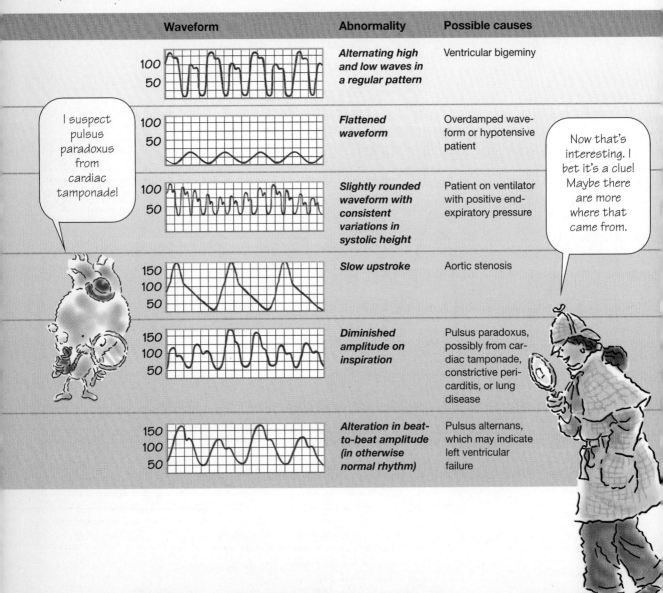

Waveform	Abnormality	Possible causes
100 50	*Alternating high and low waves in a regular pattern*	Ventricular bigeminy
100 50	*Flattened waveform*	Overdamped waveform or hypotensive patient
100 50	*Slightly rounded waveform with consistent variations in systolic height*	Patient on ventilator with positive end-expiratory pressure
150 100 50	*Slow upstroke*	Aortic stenosis
150 100 50	*Diminished amplitude on inspiration*	Pulsus paradoxus, possibly from cardiac tamponade, constrictive pericarditis, or lung disease
150 100 50	*Alteration in beat-to-beat amplitude (in otherwise normal rhythm)*	Pulsus alternans, which may indicate left ventricular failure

Pulmonary artery pressure monitoring

Continuous pulmonary artery pressure (PAP) and intermittent pulmonary artery wedge pressure (PAWP) measurements provide important information about left ventricular function and preload.

Come equipped

PA catheter

As shown here, a pulmonary artery (PA) catheter contains several lumens. Each lumen has its own purpose (indicated in parentheses).

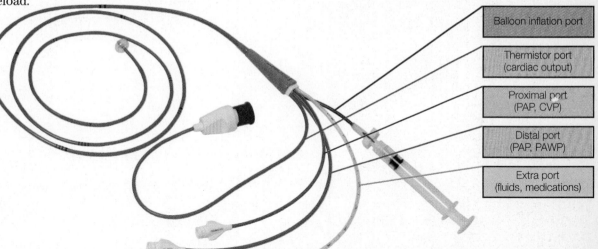

Balloon inflation port

Thermistor port (cardiac output)

Proximal port (PAP, CVP)

Distal port (PAP, PAWP)

Extra port (fluids, medications)

Normal PAP values

Right atrial pressure	1 to 6 mm Hg
Systolic right ventricular pressure	20 to 30 mm Hg
End-diastolic right ventricular pressure	Less than 5 mm Hg
Systolic PAP	20 to 30 mm Hg
Diastolic PAP	10 to 15 mm Hg
Mean PAP	Less than 20 mm Hg
PAWP	6 to 12 mm Hg

Normal pulmonary artery waveforms

After insertion into a large vein (usually the subclavian, jugular, or femoral vein), a PA catheter is advanced through the vena cava into the right atrium, through the right ventricle, and into a branch of the pulmonary artery. As the catheter advances through the heart chambers during insertion, the monitor shows various waveforms, described below.

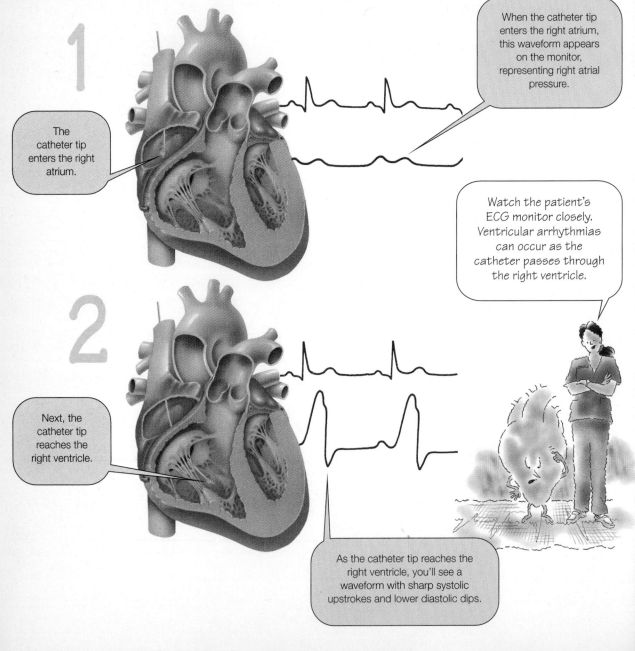

When the catheter tip enters the right atrium, this waveform appears on the monitor, representing right atrial pressure.

The catheter tip enters the right atrium.

Watch the patient's ECG monitor closely. Ventricular arrhythmias can occur as the catheter passes through the right ventricle.

Next, the catheter tip reaches the right ventricle.

As the catheter tip reaches the right ventricle, you'll see a waveform with sharp systolic upstrokes and lower diastolic dips.

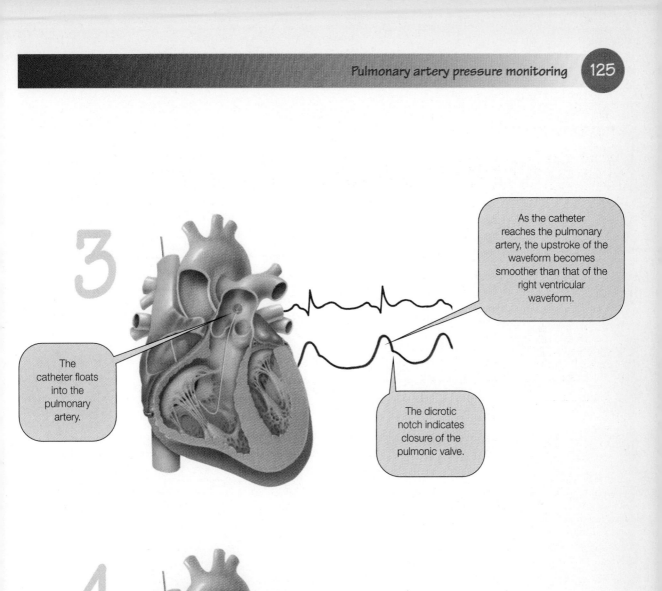

As the catheter reaches the pulmonary artery, the upstroke of the waveform becomes smoother than that of the right ventricular waveform.

The catheter floats into the pulmonary artery.

The dicrotic notch indicates closure of the pulmonic valve.

The catheter's balloon floats into a distal branch of the pulmonary artery. The balloon wedges where the vessel becomes too narrow for it to pass.

The monitor now shows a PAWP waveform with two small uprises. The balloon is then deflated and the catheter is left in the pulmonary artery.

Identifying hemodynamic pressure monitoring problems

Problem	What might cause it	What to do about it
Line fails to flush	• Inadequate pressure from pressure bag	• Make sure the pressure bag gauge reads 300 mm Hg.
	• Blood clot in catheter	• Try to aspirate the clot with a syringe. If the line still won't flush, notify the doctor and prepare to replace the line. Never use a syringe to flush a hemodynamic line.
Damped waveform	• Air bubbles	• Secure all connections. • Remove air from the lines and the transducer. • Check for and replace cracked equipment.
	• Blood flashback in line	• Make sure stopcock positions are correct; tighten loose connections and replace cracked equipment, if necessary. • Flush the line with the fast-flush valve. • Replace the transducer dome if blood backs up into it.
	• Incorrect transducer position	• Make sure the transducer is kept at the level of the right atrium at all times. Improper levels give false-high or false-low pressure readings.
	• Arterial catheter out of blood vessel or pressed against vessel wall	• Reposition the catheter if it's against the vessel wall. • Try to aspirate blood to confirm proper placement in the vessel. If you can't aspirate blood, notify the doctor and prepare to replace the line. *Note:* Bloody drainage at the insertion site may indicate catheter displacement. Notify the doctor immediately.
PAWP tracing unobtainable	• Ruptured balloon	• If you feel no resistance when injecting air or if you see blood leaking from the balloon inflation lumen, stop injecting air and notify the doctor. If the catheter is left in, label the inflation lumen with a warning not to inflate.
	• Incorrect amount of air in balloon	• Deflate the balloon. Check the label on the catheter for correct volume. Reinflate slowly with the correct amount. To avoid rupturing the balloon, never use more than the stated volume.
	• Malpositioned catheter	• Notify the doctor. Obtain a chest X-ray.

Cardiac output monitoring

Measuring cardiac output (CO)—the amount of blood ejected by the heart over 1 minute—helps evaluate cardiac function. The most widely used method for monitoring CO is the bolus thermodilution technique.

> Repeat the injection procedure at least three times to obtain a mean CO value.

photo op

Measuring cardiac output

> The injection should take no longer than 4 seconds to complete.

> When measuring cardiac output, inject the specified amount of injectant into the proximal port of the PA catheter during end expiration.

> Check the thermodilution curve on the patient's monitor to make sure that the injection was properly performed. You should see a smooth, sharp rise in the curve.

A closer look at the thermodilution method

Performed at the bedside, the thermodilution technique is the most practical method of evaluating the cardiac status of critically ill patients and those suspected of having cardiac disease. This illustration shows the path of the injectate solution through the heart during thermodilution cardiac output monitoring.

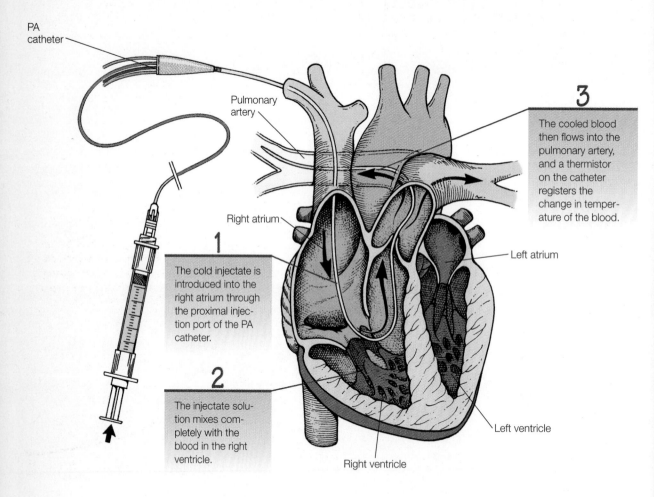

PA catheter

Pulmonary artery

Right atrium

3
The cooled blood then flows into the pulmonary artery, and a thermistor on the catheter registers the change in temperature of the blood.

Left atrium

1
The cold injectate is introduced into the right atrium through the proximal injection port of the PA catheter.

2
The injectate solution mixes completely with the blood in the right ventricle.

Left ventricle

Right ventricle

Analyzing thermodilution curves

The thermodilution curve provides valuable information about CO, injection technique, and equipment problems. When studying the curve, keep in mind that the area under the curve is inversely proportionate to CO: The smaller the area under the curve, the higher the CO; the larger the area under the curve, the lower the CO.

In addition to providing a record of CO, the curve may indicate problems related to technique, such as erratic or slow injectate instillations, or other problems, such as respiratory variations or electrical interference. The curves below correspond to those typically seen in clinical practice.

Normal thermodilution curve

In a patient who has adequate CO, the thermodilution curve begins with a smooth, rapid upstroke (representing proper injection technique) and is followed by a smooth, gradual downslope. The height of the curve varies, depending on whether you use a room-temperature or an iced injectate.

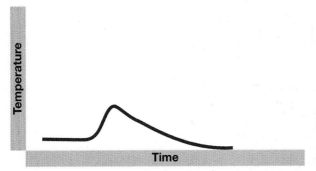

High CO curve

A high CO curve has a rapid, smooth upstroke. Because the ventricles are ejecting blood too forcefully, the injectate moves through the heart quickly and the curve returns to baseline more rapidly. The smaller area under the curve suggests high CO.

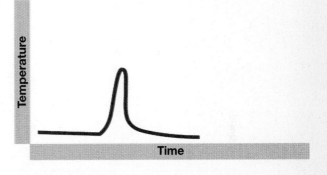

Low CO curve

A low CO curve has a rapid, smooth upstroke. However, because blood is being ejected less efficiently from the ventricles, the injectate warms slowly and takes longer to be ejected. Consequently, the curve takes longer to return to baseline. This slow return produces a larger area under the curve, corresponding to low CO.

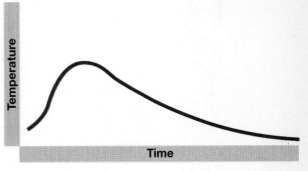

Cardiac index

* Measurement of CO per unit of time that takes into account the patient's body surface area (BSA)

* Normally calculated in L/minute/m²

$$\text{Cardiac index} = CO \div BSA$$

Normal ranges

For nonpregnant adults: 2.5 to 4.2 L/minute/m²

For pregnant women: 3.5 to 6.5 L/minute/m²

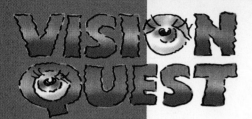

Able to label?

Label each component of the normal arterial waveform shown here.

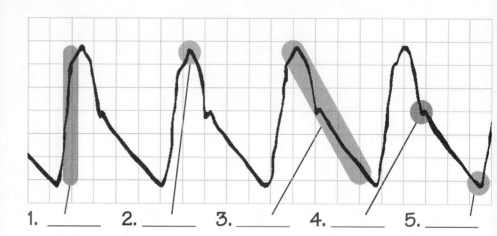

1. _____ 2. _____ 3. _____ 4. _____ 5. _____

Matchmaker

Match the abnormal arterial waveforms shown to their possible causes.

1.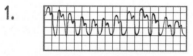

2.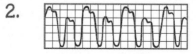

3.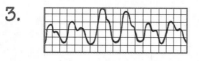

4.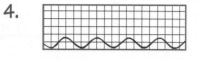

5.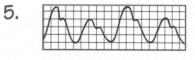

6.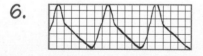

A. Pulsus paradoxus

B. Ventilator

C. Pulsus alternans

D. Ventricular bigeminy

E. Aortic stenosis

F. Overdamped waveform

6 Common disorders

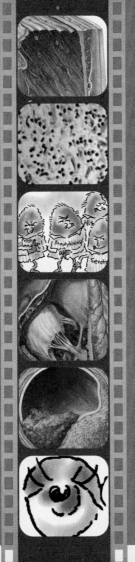

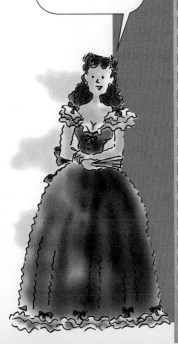

Woe is me! With such a complicated system, so many things can go wrong.

Inflammatory disorders

Inflammatory cardiac disorders include endocarditis, myocarditis, and pericarditis. In patients with these conditions, scar formation and otherwise normal healing processes can cause debilitating structural damage to the heart.

Endocarditis

Endocarditis is an inflammation of the endocardium, the heart valves, or a cardiac prosthesis. It typically results from bacterial invasion and, therefore, may also be referred to as *infective endocarditis (IE)*.

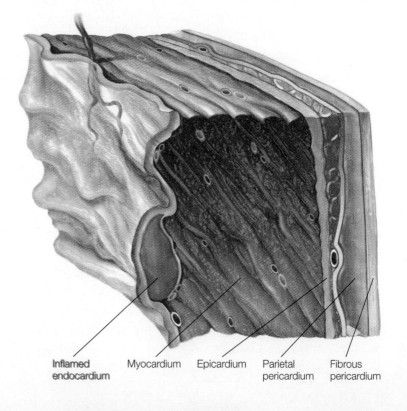

Inflamed endocardium   Myocardium   Epicardium   Parietal pericardium   Fibrous pericardium

Libman-Sacks endocarditis

Found in patients with systemic lupus erythematosus, Libman-Sacks endocarditis is characterized by wartlike vegetations on the leaflets of the mitral valve.

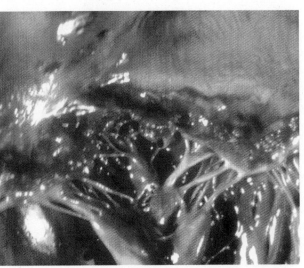

Untreated endocarditis usually proves fatal. However, with proper treatment, 70% of patients recover.

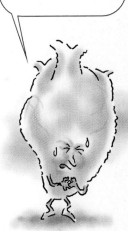

Bacterial endocarditis

In bacterial endocarditis, the leaflets of the mitral valve erode and are eventually destroyed by bacterial invasion.

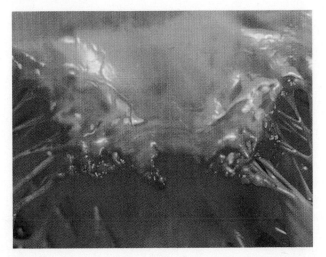

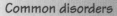

What's in a name?

The terminology used to describe IE changes as the causes of the disease become better understood. Some common names include:

■ **acute IE**—describes a rapidly progressive disease process
■ **subacute IE**—describes a disease process that lasts several months
■ **rheumatic IE**—describes disease caused by rheumatic fever–related damage to heart valves.

New names on the IE scene include:

■ **native valve IE**—affects original heart valves
■ **prosthetic valve IE**—affects artificial heart valves
■ **IVDA IE**—affects I.V. drug abusers
■ **nosocomial IE**—describes disease that's associated with hospitalization.

Signs and symptoms of endocarditis

■ Weakness and fatigue
■ Anorexia
■ Arthralgia
■ Intermittent fever
■ Loud, regurgitant murmur

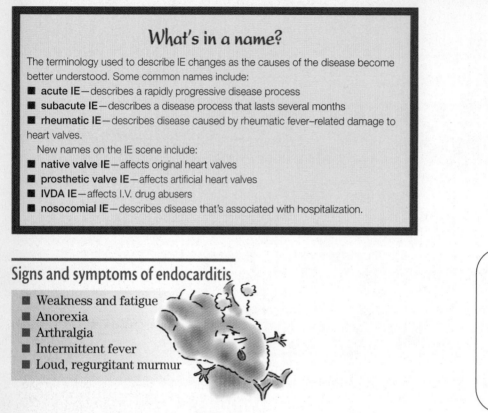

Treatment of endocarditis seeks to eradicate the infecting organisms. Common organisms include staphylococci, especially *S. aureus*, streptococci, and *Candida albicans*.

℞
■ I.V. antibiotics
■ Oral antibiotics
■ Corrective surgery

Myocarditis

Myocarditis is focal or diffuse inflammation of the cardiac muscle (myocardium). It can be acute or chronic and can occur at any age.

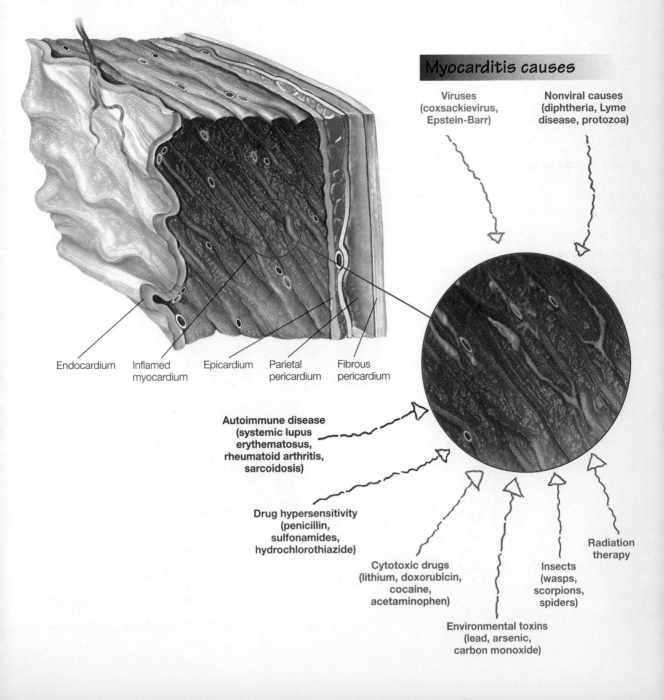

Endocardium

Inflamed myocardium

Epicardium

Parietal pericardium

Fibrous pericardium

Myocarditis causes

Viruses (coxsackievirus, Epstein-Barr)

Nonviral causes (diphtheria, Lyme disease, protozoa)

Autoimmune disease (systemic lupus erythematosus, rheumatoid arthritis, sarcoidosis)

Drug hypersensitivity (penicillin, sulfonamides, hydrochlorothiazide)

Cytotoxic drugs (lithium, doxorubicin, cocaine, acetaminophen)

Environmental toxins (lead, arsenic, carbon monoxide)

Insects (wasps, scorpions, spiders)

Radiation therapy

Viral myocarditis

Viral infections are the most common cause of myocarditis in the United States.

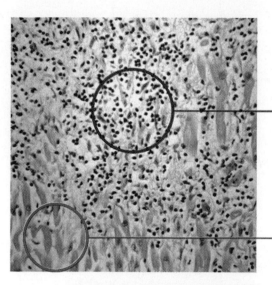

Lymphocytes and macrophages invade the myocardial muscle fibers, force them apart, and disrupt their normal function.

Normal myocardial fibers

Signs and symptoms of myocarditis

- Dyspnea and fatigue
- Palpitations
- Fever
- Mild, continuous pressure or soreness in the chest
- Signs and symptoms of heart failure (with severe disease)

Usually...

Myocarditis fails to produce specific cardiovascular symptoms or ECG abnormalities. The patient commonly experiences spontaneous recovery without residual defects.

Sometimes...

The myocardium becomes damaged. As a result, arrhythmias, left-sided heart enlargement, and scarring can occur, but these problems can usually be readily managed.

Rarely...

Myocarditis is complicated by heart failure and leads to cardiomyopathy or arrhythmia-related death.

Rx

- Modified bed rest (up to 6 months)
- I.V. immune globulin drugs
- Management of complications

Pericarditis

Pericarditis is an inflammation of the pericardium. Although it's sometimes idiopathic, common causes of pericarditis include infection, radiation therapy, and myocardial infarction (MI).

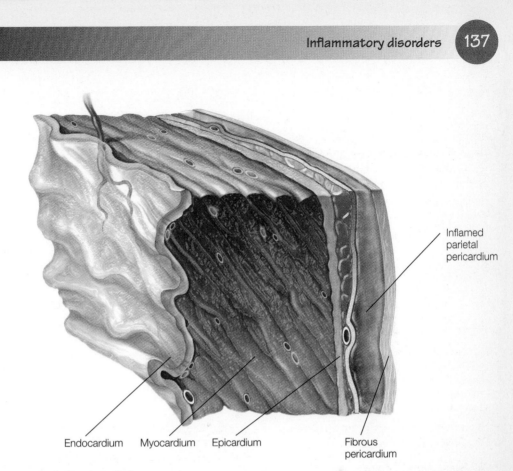

Inflamed parietal pericardium

Endocardium   Myocardium   Epicardium   Fibrous pericardium

The inflammatory process in pericarditis

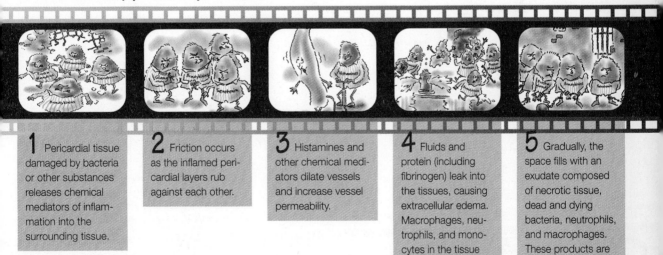

1 Pericardial tissue damaged by bacteria or other substances releases chemical mediators of inflammation into the surrounding tissue.

2 Friction occurs as the inflamed pericardial layers rub against each other.

3 Histamines and other chemical mediators dilate vessels and increase vessel permeability.

4 Fluids and protein (including fibrinogen) leak into the tissues, causing extracellular edema. Macrophages, neutrophils, and monocytes in the tissue begin to phagocytose the invading bacteria.

5 Gradually, the space fills with an exudate composed of necrotic tissue, dead and dying bacteria, neutrophils, and macrophages. These products are eventually reabsorbed into healthy tissue.

Acute

Acute pericarditis can be fibrinous or effusive with purulent, serous, or hemorrhagic exudate. Buildup of fluid can cause pericardial effusion. If the effusion builds too rapidly, cardiac tamponade may occur.

Signs and symptoms of acute pericarditis

Sharp, sudden pain, usually starting over the sternum and radiating to the neck, shoulders, back, and arms

Pericardial friction rub at left third intercostal space

Chronic

Chronic constrictive pericarditis is characterized by dense, fibrous pericardial thickening (shown below). This thickening causes constriction of normal heart size and movement, which can lead to permanently reduced stroke volume and cardiac output.

Signs and symptoms of chronic constrictive pericarditis

- Dyspnea
- Fatigue
- Chest pain with exertion
- Inspiratory jugular vein distention (Kussmaul's sign)
- Ascites and peripheral edema

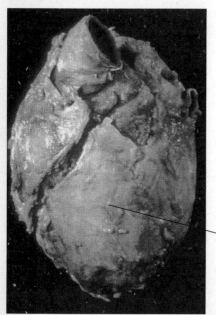

Thick, fibrous pericardium

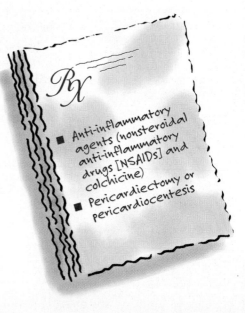

Rx

- Anti-inflammatory agents (nonsteroidal anti-inflammatory drugs [NSAIDs] and colchicine)
- Pericardiectomy or pericardiocentesis

Valvular disorders

Valvular disease, which can occur in any of the heart valves, can be characterized as prolapse, insufficiency, or stenosis. It causes problems with opening and closing of the valves.

Possible causes

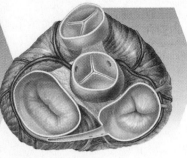

- Myxomatous degeneration (weakening with aging)
- Calcific degeneration
- IE
- Coronary artery disease (CAD)
- MI

Potential complications

- Arrhythmias
- Cardiomyopathy
- Heart failure
- Thrombotic disorders

Mitral valve prolapse

Generally a benign disorder, mitral valve prolapse is often called *click-murmur syndrome* because of the auscultatory sounds commonly associated with it. Some patients complain of palpitations or chest pain.

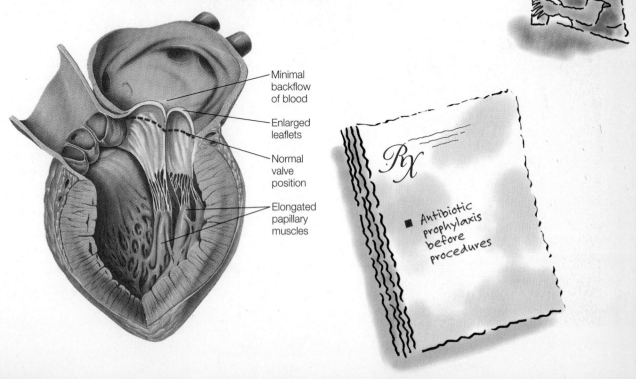

- Minimal backflow of blood
- Enlarged leaflets
- Normal valve position
- Elongated papillary muscles

℞

- Antibiotic prophylaxis before procedures

Mitral insufficiency

Mitral insufficiency occurs when the mitral valve doesn't close completely, allowing blood to flow back through the valve.

1 Blood from the left ventricle flows back into the left atrium during systole, causing the atrium to enlarge to accommodate the backflow.

2 As a result, the left ventricle dilates to accommodate the increased blood volume from the atrium and to compensate for diminished cardiac output.

3 Ventricular hypertrophy and increased back pressure in the left atrium result in increased pulmonary artery pressure, eventually leading to left-sided and right-sided heart failure.

You'll hear a holosystolic murmur if you listen at the apex of the heart.

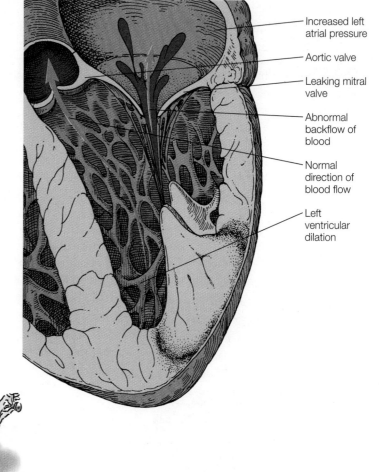

Increased left atrial pressure

Aortic valve

Leaking mitral valve

Abnormal backflow of blood

Normal direction of blood flow

Left ventricular dilation

Acute

Acute mitral insufficiency can start suddenly, with the characteristic sign being severe dyspnea.

Chronic

Chronic mitral insufficiency is a slow process that's accompanied by symptoms such as fatigue and insomnia.

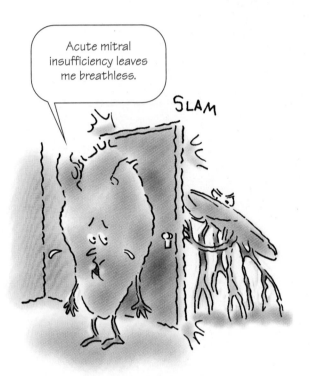

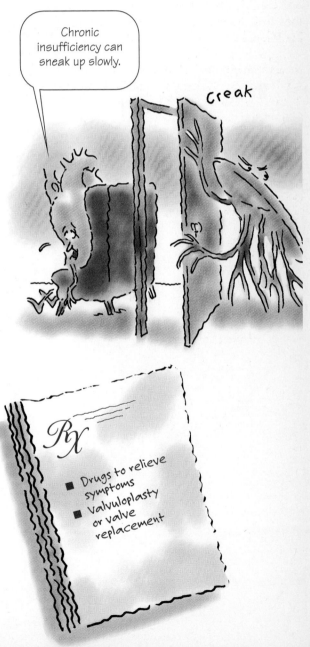

Signs and symptoms

- Orthopnea or dyspnea
- Fatigue
- Angina and palpitations
- New-onset atrial fibrillation
- Systolic murmur

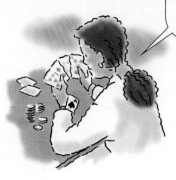

Call it lady luck. Mitral stenosis typically occurs in females. It most commonly results from rheumatic fever and may also be associated with congenital anomalies.

Mitral valve stenosis

Mitral valve stenosis is hardening of the mitral valve caused by fibrosis or calcification. This hardening results in narrowing of the valve opening, which obstructs blood flow from the left atrium to the left ventricle. Consequently, left atrial volume and pressure increase and the chamber dilates.

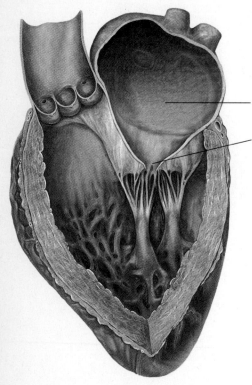

Pulmonary hypertension develops

Left atrium dilation

Narrowed mitral valve

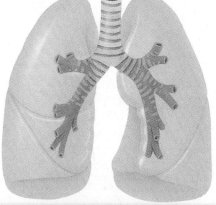

Lung congestion and pressure

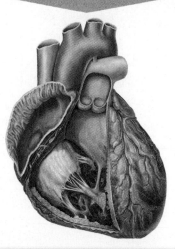

Right-sided heart failure

Signs and symptoms

■ Dyspnea on exertion, paroxysmal nocturnal dyspnea, and orthopnea
■ Fatigue and weakness
■ Right-sided heart failure and cardiac arrhythmias
■ Crackles on auscultation

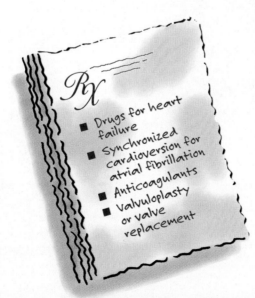

I get all choked up when your mitral valve narrows and you start acting really irregular.

Yeah, well, I really fibrillate when my left atrium enlarges and stretches my conduction fibers. Sorry the pressure comes back on you.

℞

■ Drugs for heart failure
■ Synchronized cardioversion for atrial fibrillation
■ Anticoagulants
■ Valvuloplasty or valve replacement

Aortic insufficiency

Aortic insufficiency occurs when the aortic semilunar valve doesn't close completely. In this condition, blood flows back through the valve into the left ventricle. It can result from rheumatic fever, syphilis, hypertension, or endocarditis, or it may be idiopathic. It's also associated with Marfan syndrome and with ventricular septal defect, even after surgical closure.

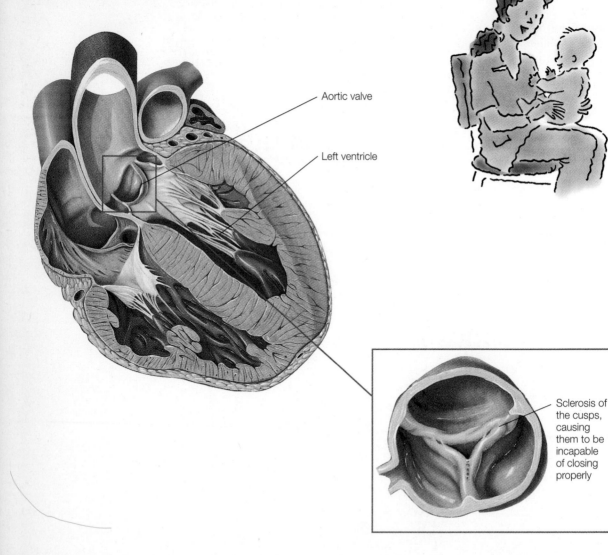

Oh boy. Aortic insufficiency typically occurs in males.

Aortic valve

Left ventricle

Sclerosis of the cusps, causing them to be incapable of closing properly

Signs and symptoms

- Exertional dyspnea
- Cough
- Left-sided heart failure
- Pulsus bisferiens (rapidly rising and collapsing pulses)
- Blowing diastolic murmur or S_3

A sign by any other name...

Many common signs seen in aortic insufficiency have been named after the physicians who first documented them. Here are a few for you to spot.

Sign	Description
de Musset's sign	Bobbing of the head with every pulse
Hill's sign	Blood pressure that's higher in the arms than in the legs
Quincke's sign	Pulsatile flushing and blanching of the fingernail bed with gentle pressure
Traube's sign	Pistol-shot-like sound auscultated over the femoral arteries

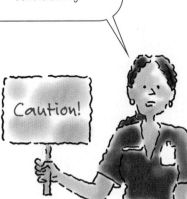

Patients with aortic insufficiency are rarely treated with beta blockers due to these drugs' negative effects on myocardial contractility.

Caution!

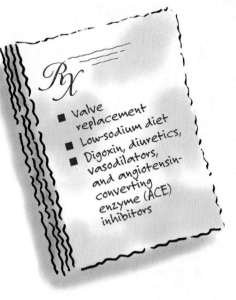

Rx

- Valve replacement
- Low-sodium diet
- Digoxin, diuretics, vasodilators, and angiotensin-converting enzyme (ACE) inhibitors

Aortic stenosis

Aortic stenosis results from a congenital aortic valve defect, congenital stenosis of valve cusps, or rheumatic fever.

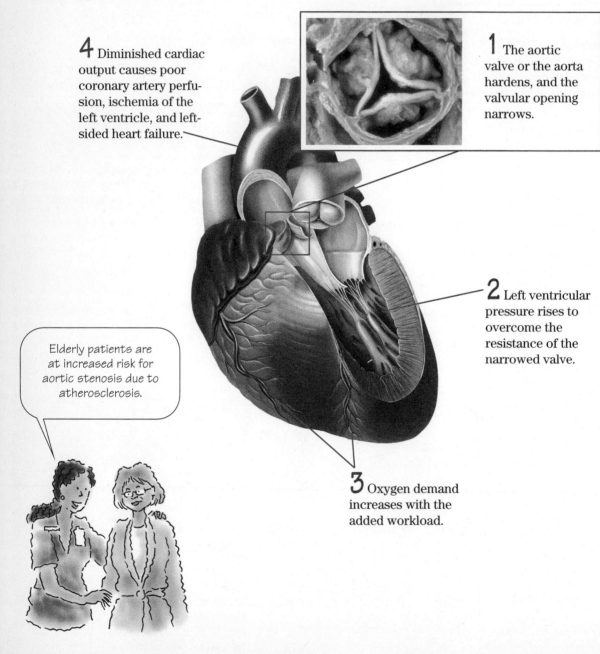

4 Diminished cardiac output causes poor coronary artery perfusion, ischemia of the left ventricle, and left-sided heart failure.

1 The aortic valve or the aorta hardens, and the valvular opening narrows.

2 Left ventricular pressure rises to overcome the resistance of the narrowed valve.

Elderly patients are at increased risk for aortic stenosis due to atherosclerosis.

3 Oxygen demand increases with the added workload.

Signs and symptoms

■ Exertional dyspnea and paroxysmal nocturnal dyspnea
■ Syncope
■ Angina, palpitations, and cardiac arrhythmias
■ Left-sided heart failure
■ Systolic murmur at the base of the carotids

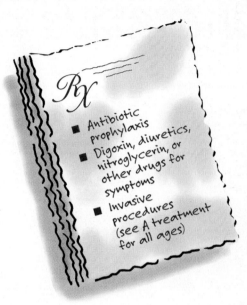

Rx
■ Antibiotic prophylaxis
■ Digoxin, diuretics, or nitroglycerin, or other drugs for symptoms
■ Invasive procedures (see A treatment for all ages)

A treatment for all ages

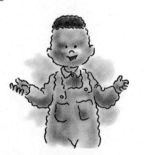

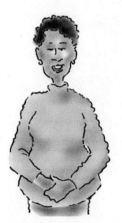

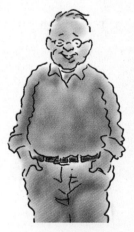

In children who don't have calcified valves, simple commissurotomy under direct visualization is usually effective.

Adults with calcified valves need valve replacement when they become symptomatic or are at risk for developing left-sided heart failure.

Percutaneous balloon aortic valvuloplasty is useful in elderly patients with severe calcifications and in children and young adults who have congenital aortic stenosis. This procedure may improve left ventricular function so that the patient can tolerate valve replacement surgery.

Degenerative disorders

Degenerative disorders, which cause damage over time, are the most common cardiovascular ailments. The onset of these disorders may be insidious, triggering symptoms only after the disease has progressed.

Hypertension

Hypertension refers to intermittent or sustained elevation in diastolic or systolic blood pressure (BP).

Types of hypertension and their causes

Essential (primary, idiopathic)

- Caused by complex abnormalities in the mechanisms that control cardiac output, systemic vascular resistance, and blood volume
- More than 90% of all cases

Causes

- Environmental factors, such as obesity, stress, and high salt intake
- Genetic factors, such as insulin resistance
- Increased sympathetic nervous system activity

Secondary

- Caused by another disorder
- Less than 10% of all cases

Causes

- Renovascular diseases or primary aldosteronism
- Congenital coarctation (narrowing) of the aorta
- Hormonal contraceptives
- Sleep apnea

Signs and symptoms

- Increased BP measurements on two or more readings taken at two or more visits after an initial screening
- Throbbing occipital headaches with vision problems upon waking
- Drowsiness
- Evidence of disease causing secondary hypertension
- Complications of sustained elevation

> Malignant hypertension is a rare, severe form of hypertension that's characterized by a BP of 220/120 mm Hg or more.

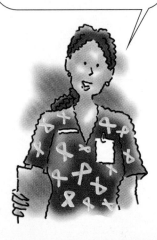

Blood pressure classifications

BP is also classified based on the degree of elevation of the readings. This table classifies blood pressure according to systolic blood pressure (SBP) and diastolic blood pressure (DBP).

BP classification	Normal	Prehypertension	Stage 1	Stage 2
SBP (mm Hg)	< 120 and	120 to 139 or	140 to 159 or	≥ 160 or
DBP (mm Hg)	< 80	80 to 89	90 to 99	≥ 100

The silent killer

Although patients may feel healthy, untreated or poorly controlled hypertension can be damaging to their major organs.

Brain

Stroke

Stroke from blood clots in narrowed blood vessels or from hemorrhage of a weakened vessel wall (aneurysm) can be disabling or fatal.

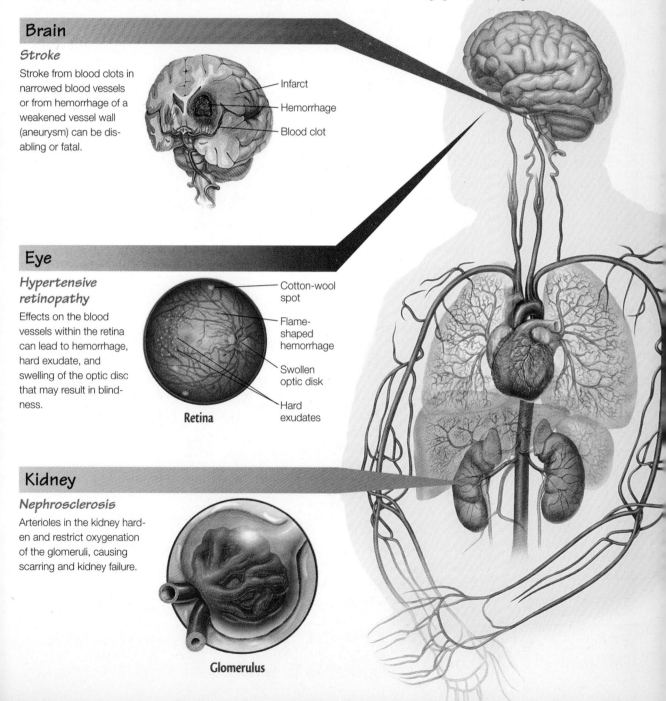

Infarct

Hemorrhage

Blood clot

Eye

Hypertensive retinopathy

Effects on the blood vessels within the retina can lead to hemorrhage, hard exudate, and swelling of the optic disc that may result in blindness.

Cotton-wool spot

Flame-shaped hemorrhage

Swollen optic disk

Hard exudates

Retina

Kidney

Nephrosclerosis

Arterioles in the kidney harden and restrict oxygenation of the glomeruli, causing scarring and kidney failure.

Glomerulus

Preventing pressure problems

Preventing the onset of hypertension is the first goal of the Joint National Committee on Prevention, Detection, Evaluation, and Treatment of High Blood Pressure. Evidence shows that lifestyle interventions, such as those listed here, are critical to meeting this goal:

- increasing exercise
- consuming a diet that's low in salt, fat, and cholesterol
- maintaining a body mass index < 30
- limiting alcohol intake.

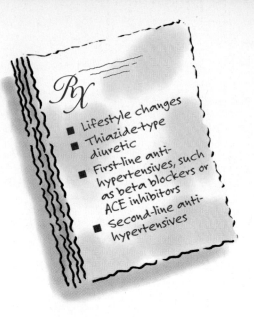

Pulmonary hypertension

Pulmonary hypertension refers to chronically elevated pulmonary artery pressure (PAP) over 30 mm Hg and a mean PAP over 20 mm Hg plus increased pulmonary vascular resistance.

There are two types of pulmonary hypertension:
- In *primary*, or *idiopathic*, pulmonary hypertension, the intimal linings of the pulmonary arteries thicken, narrowing the lumen and increasing vascular resistance. No cause is known.
- *Secondary* pulmonary hypertension begins with diseases that cause alveolar destruction or prevent the chest wall from expanding sufficiently.

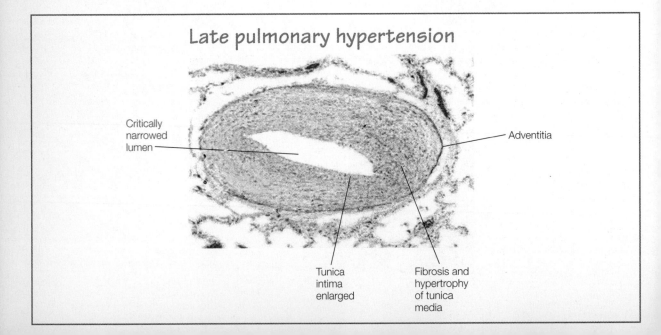

Late pulmonary hypertension

Critically narrowed lumen

Adventitia

Tunica intima enlarged

Fibrosis and hypertrophy of tunica media

What happens?

Pulmonary hypertension can be caused by a number of factors, all of which force the heart's right side to work harder to pump blood to the lungs. The right chambers may enlarge as they struggle to function, and blood is often forced backward through the tricuspid valve.

Signs and symptoms

- Exertional dyspnea, weakness, syncope, and fatigue
- Tachycardia
- Decreased BP
- Tachypnea with mild exertion
- Changes in mental status, from restlessness to agitation or confusion
- Easily palpable right ventricular lift and a reduced carotid pulse

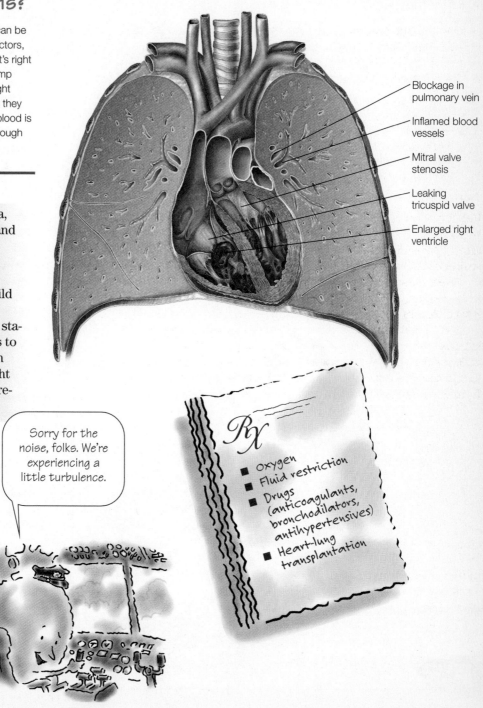

Blockage in pulmonary vein

Inflamed blood vessels

Mitral valve stenosis

Leaking tricuspid valve

Enlarged right ventricle

Sorry for the noise, folks. We're experiencing a little turbulence.

℞
- Oxygen
- Fluid restriction
- Drugs (anticoagulants, bronchodilators, antihypertensives)
- Heart-lung transplantation

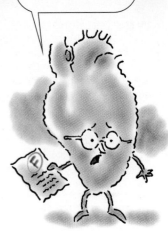

They say I'm a failure! But it's not my fault.

Heart failure

Heart failure occurs when the myocardium can't pump effectively enough to meet the body's metabolic needs. A complex interaction of the factors listed here leads to the syndrome of heart failure:

■ altered myocardial function due to increased pressure or volume within the heart

■ left ventricular remodeling, with initial hypertrophy and then severe dilation

■ altered hemodynamics that result from an effort to maintain cardiac output despite increased diastolic filling pressure

■ neurohormonal changes that accelerate heart rate and initially increase ejection fraction, then trigger a local inflammatory response that becomes systemic in severe disease.

Left ventricular hypertrophy

Hypertrophy of the left ventricle is one of the heart's first steps to compensate for either increased pressures or increased blood volume.

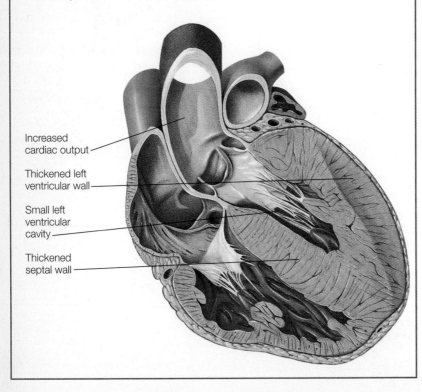

Increased cardiac output

Thickened left ventricular wall

Small left ventricular cavity

Thickened septal wall

A Starling named Frank?

The Frank-Starling law says that the amount of cardiac muscle stretch correlates directly with the force of contraction. This accounts for the heart's ability to pump more blood during exertion in addition to its ability to compensate for sustained abnormal increases in blood volume.

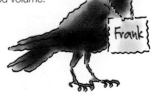

Three ways to classify heart failure

Heart failure can be classified according to its pathophysiology. It may be right-sided or left-sided, systolic or diastolic, and acute or chronic.

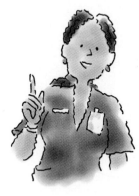

1 Right-sided or left-sided

Right-sided heart failure is the result of ineffective right ventricular contraction. It may be caused by an acute right ventricular infarction or pulmonary embolus. However, the most common cause is profound backward blood flow due to left-sided heart failure.

Left-sided heart failure is the result of ineffective left ventricular contraction. It may lead to pulmonary congestion or pulmonary edema and decreased cardiac output. Left ventricular MI, hypertension, and aortic or mitral valve stenosis or insufficiency are common causes. As the left ventricle's decreased pumping ability persists, fluid accumulates, backing up into the left atrium, then into the lungs. If this worsens, pulmonary edema and right-sided heart failure may also result.

2 Systolic or diastolic

In systolic heart failure, the left ventricle can't pump enough blood out to the systemic circulation during systole and the ejection fraction falls. Consequently, blood backs up into the pulmonary circulation, pressure rises in the pulmonary venous system, and cardiac output falls.

In diastolic heart failure, the left ventricle can't relax and fill properly during diastole and the stroke volume falls. Therefore, larger ventricular volumes are needed to maintain cardiac output.

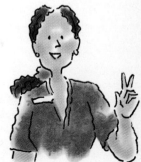

3 Acute or chronic

The term *acute* refers to the timing of the onset of symptoms and whether compensatory mechanisms kick in. Typically, in acute heart failure, fluid status is normal or low, and sodium and water retention don't occur.

In chronic heart failure, signs and symptoms have been present for some time, compensatory mechanisms have taken effect, and fluid volume overload persists. Drugs, diet changes, and activity restrictions usually control symptoms.

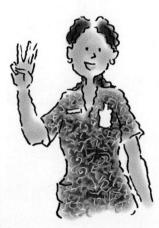

Signs and symptoms of right-sided failure

- Edema, initially dependent
- Jugular vein distention
- Hepatomegaly
- Generalized weight gain

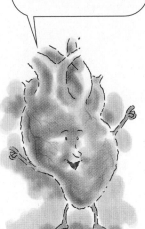

Who knew my split personality could have such an effect on the body?

Signs and symptoms of left-sided failure

- Dyspnea, initially on exertion
- Cough
- Tachycardia
- Fatigue
- Muscle weakness
- Edema and weight gain
- Bibasilar crackles

photo op

Looking for edema

Compare one foot and leg with the other, noting their relative size and the prominence of veins, tendons, and bones. Note that edema may obscure these features. Edema can be pitting or nonpitting.

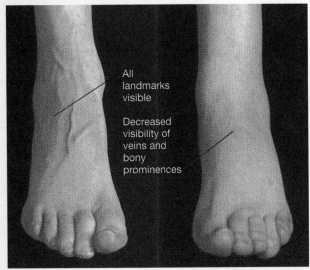

All landmarks visible

Decreased visibility of veins and bony prominences

Normal   Edematous

Pitting edema

"Pitting" is a result of the inelasticity of fluid-filled tissue. To differentiate pitting edema from nonpitting edema, press your finger against a swollen area for 5 seconds and then quickly remove it. If the indentation fills slowly, pitting edema is present. To determine the severity of pitting edema, estimate the indentation's depth in centimeters: +1 (1 cm), +2 (2 cm), +3 (3 cm), or +4 (4 cm).

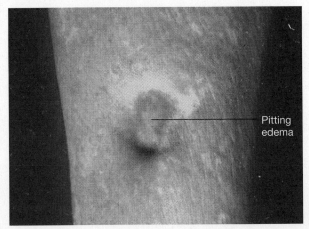

Pitting edema

Classifying signs and symptoms to determine treatment

Two sets of guidelines are available to help direct treatment of patients with heart failure. The New York Heart Association (NYHA) classification is based on functional capacity. The American College of Cardiology/American Heart Association (ACC/AHA) guidelines are based on objective assessment. These guidelines are compared side-by-side below.

NYHA classification	ACC/AHA guidelines	Recommendations
	Stage A: Patient at high risk for developing heart failure but without structural heart disease or signs and symptoms of heart failure	▪ Treatment of hypertension, lipid disorders, and diabetes ▪ Smoking cessation and regular exercise ▪ Discouraged use of alcohol and illicit drugs ▪ Angiotensin-converting enzyme (ACE) inhibitor, if indicated
Class I: Ordinary physical activity doesn't cause undue fatigue, palpitations, dyspnea, or angina.	**Stage B:** Structural heart disease without signs and symptoms of heart failure	▪ All stage A therapies ▪ ACE inhibitor (unless contraindicated) ▪ Beta-adrenergic blocker (unless contraindicated)
Class II: Patient has slight limitation of physical activity but is asymptomatic at rest. Ordinary physical activity causes fatigue, palpitations, dyspnea, or anginal pain. **Class III:** Patient has marked limitation of physical activity but is typically asymptomatic at rest. Less than ordinary physical activity causes fatigue, palpitations, dyspnea, or angina.	**Stage C:** Structural heart disease with prior or current signs and symptoms of heart failure	▪ All stage A and B therapies ▪ Sodium-restricted diet ▪ Diuretics ▪ Digoxin ▪ Avoiding or withdrawing antiarrhythmic agents, most calcium channel blockers, and NSAIDs ▪ Drug therapy, including aldosterone antagonists, angiotensin receptor blockers, hydralazine, and nitrates
Class IV: Patient is unable to perform any physical activity without discomfort; symptoms may be present at rest. Discomfort increases with physical activity.	**Stage D:** End-stage disease requiring specialized treatment strategies, such as mechanical circulatory support, continuous inotropic infusion, or heart transplantation	▪ All therapies for stages A, B, and C ▪ Mechanical assist device, such as biventricular pacemaker or left ventricular assist device ▪ Continuous inotropic therapy ▪ Hospice care

Rx

▪ Treatment of underlying disorders
▪ Lifestyle changes to decrease effects
▪ Drugs per protocol above
▪ Ventricular assist device or heart transplantation

A smaller "dor"

The Dor procedure, also called *partial left ventriculectomy* or *ventricular remodeling*, involves the removal of nonviable heart muscle to reduce the size of the hypertrophied ventricle, thereby allowing the heart to pump more efficiently. This procedure isn't indicated for all patients, though.

Cardiomyopathy

Cardiomyopathy generally refers to disease of the heart muscle fibers. It takes three main forms.

Dilated cardiomyopathy

Dilated cardiomyopathy primarily affects systolic function. Here's what happens:

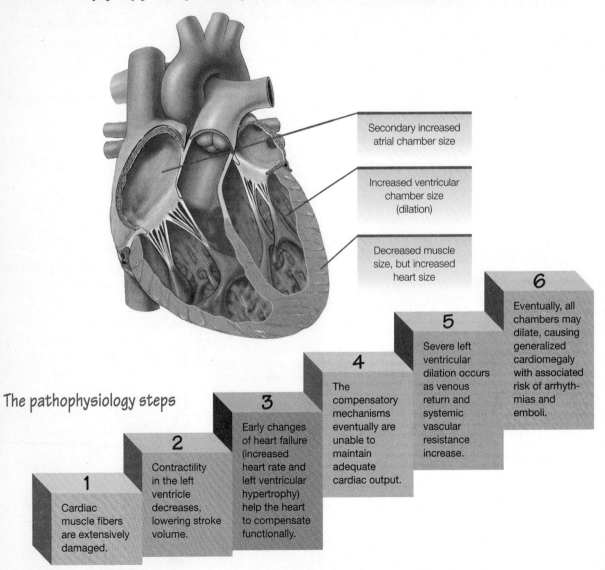

Secondary increased atrial chamber size

Increased ventricular chamber size (dilation)

Decreased muscle size, but increased heart size

The pathophysiology steps

1 Cardiac muscle fibers are extensively damaged.

2 Contractility in the left ventricle decreases, lowering stroke volume.

3 Early changes of heart failure (increased heart rate and left ventricular hypertrophy) help the heart to compensate functionally.

4 The compensatory mechanisms eventually are unable to maintain adequate cardiac output.

5 Severe left ventricular dilation occurs as venous return and systemic vascular resistance increase.

6 Eventually, all chambers may dilate, causing generalized cardiomegaly with associated risk of arrhythmias and emboli.

Signs and symptoms

■ Shortness of breath, orthopnea, dyspnea on exertion, paroxysmal nocturnal dyspnea, fatigue, and a dry cough at night caused by left-sided heart failure
■ Peripheral edema, hepatomegaly, jugular vein distention, and weight gain caused by right-sided heart failure
■ Tachycardia with irregular pulse, if atrial fibrillation exists
■ Pansystolic murmur associated with mitral and tricuspid insufficiency

For a patient with dilated cardiomyopathy, signs and symptoms may be overlooked until left-sided heart failure occurs. Evaluate the patient's current condition; then compare it with his condition over the past 6 to 12 months.

Rx
■ Treatment of underlying disorders
■ Lifestyle modifications to increase functional capacity
■ ACE inhibitors
■ Drugs to treat heart failure and arrhythmias
■ Heart transplantation

Hypertrophic cardiomyopathy

Hypertrophic cardiomyopathy primarily affects diastolic function. Here's what happens:

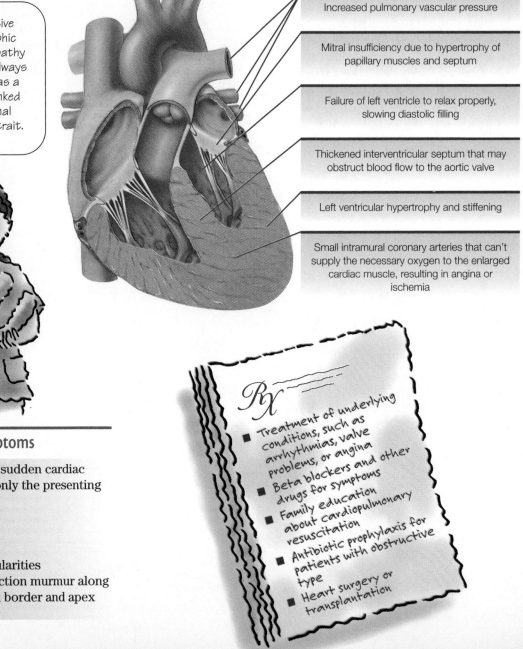

Obstructive hypertrophic cardiomyopathy is almost always inherited as a non-sex-linked autosomal dominant trait.

Increased pulmonary vascular pressure

Mitral insufficiency due to hypertrophy of papillary muscles and septum

Failure of left ventricle to relax properly, slowing diastolic filling

Thickened interventricular septum that may obstruct blood flow to the aortic valve

Left ventricular hypertrophy and stiffening

Small intramural coronary arteries that can't supply the necessary oxygen to the enlarged cardiac muscle, resulting in angina or ischemia

Signs and symptoms

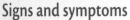

- Syncope or sudden cardiac death (commonly the presenting symptom)
- Angina
- Dyspnea
- Fatigue
- Pulse irregularities
- Systolic ejection murmur along the left sternal border and apex

R_x
- Treatment of underlying conditions, such as arrhythmias, valve problems, or angina
- Beta blockers and other drugs for symptoms
- Family education about cardiopulmonary resuscitation
- Antibiotic prophylaxis for patients with obstructive type
- Heart surgery or transplantation

Restrictive cardiomyopathy

Restrictive cardiomyopathy is characterized by stiffness of the ventricle caused by left ventricular hypertrophy and endocardial fibrosis and thickening. Here's what happens:

Decreased cardiac output with high diastolic pressure compared to the amount of diastolic volume

Enlarged atria due to rigid ventricular walls, causing atrial fibrillation

Failure of the left ventricle to relax properly, slowing diastolic filling

Mild to no left ventricular hypertrophy

Ventricular rigidity from fibrosis that impairs contraction during systole

Incompetent atrioventricular valves, allowing backward flow of blood

Decreased ventricular chamber size from endocardial fibrosis and thickening

Signs and symptoms

- Fatigue
- Dyspnea
- Orthopnea
- Chest pain
- Edema
- Liver engorgement
- High systemic and pulmonary venous pressure

Keep an eye out: restrictive cardiomyopathy can resemble constrictive pericarditis.

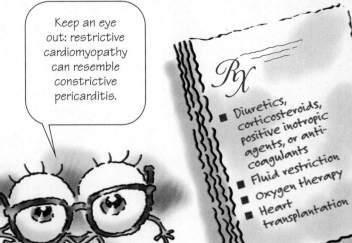

Rx
- Diuretics, corticosteroids, positive inotropic agents, or anti-coagulants
- Fluid restriction
- Oxygen therapy
- Heart transplantation

Coronary artery disease

CAD results from the progressive buildup of atherosclerotic plaque in the coronary arteries.

The law of supply and demand

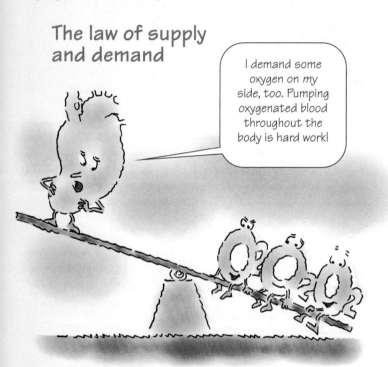

I demand some oxygen on my side, too. Pumping oxygenated blood throughout the body is hard work!

---

memory board

CAD risk factors

To remember the risk factors for CAD, just think about the word **RISKS:**

Rising LDL and triglyceride levels—LDLs should be < 130 mg/dl, triglycerides < 200 mg/dl.

Inadequate control of hypertension, diabetes, and obesity—Diet and exercise lifestyle changes are the first step to regaining control.

Sex—CAD is more common in men until after age 75.

Kinfolk—Heredity is a nonmodifiable risk factor.

Smoking—The sooner stopped, the better.

Coronary artery close-up

Coronary arteries are normally flexible and can adapt to the oxygen-carrying needs of the heart.

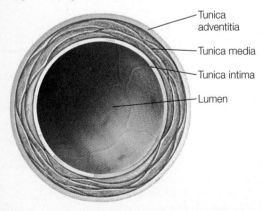

- Tunica adventitia
- Tunica media
- Tunica intima
- Lumen

Understanding atherosclerosis

Atherosclerosis causes a buildup of fatty fibrous plaque in the vessel walls. Thrombi can also form if the plaque ruptures through the intimal layer. The lumen becomes increasingly narrow.

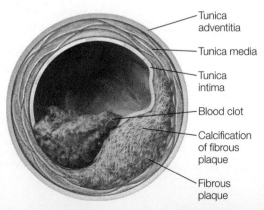

- Tunica adventitia
- Tunica media
- Tunica intima
- Blood clot
- Calcification of fibrous plaque
- Fibrous plaque

Signs and symptoms

- Possibly none
- Abnormal stress or echocardiogram findings
- Angina, typically with exertion or stress
- Major complications, such as acute coronary syndrome, heart failure, arrhythmias, or sudden death

Did you know I can cause mitral insufficiency and cardiomyopathy, too?

Stable angina

Angina is the classic sign of CAD. Stable angina can come in three forms: Prinzmetal's (variant) angina, microvascular (cardiac syndrome X) angina, and chronic stable angina.

Partially blocked artery, causing chronic stable angina

Capillary constriction, causing microvascular angina without blockage of coronary arteries

Area of vasospasm, causing Prinzmetal's angina

Prinzmetal's (variant) angina

- Characterized by resting discomfort, which can cause the patient to awaken at night and persists for hours
- Causes reversible ST-segment elevation during event
- Caused by coronary artery vasospasm
- Treated with calcium channel blockers and nitrates, possibly beta blockers, or coronary stenting if intractable

Microvascular (cardiac syndrome X) angina

- Characterized by stable, angina-like chest pain
- Caused by impairment of vasodilator reserve
- Poses no risk of cardiac ischemia because the capillaries are too small to block oxygenation of cardiac cells
- Treated with nitrates, beta blockers, or calcium channel blockers

Chronic stable angina

- Characterized by exertional, rest-relieved discomfort located anywhere between the umbilicus and the ears that may be associated with numbness of the arms or hands
- Doesn't increase in frequency or severity over time
- Generally caused by fixed obstructive atheromatous lesions
- Treated with rest and nitrates; beta blockers for prevention

Acute coronary syndromes

Patients with acute coronary syndromes (ACS) have some degree of coronary artery occlusion. Development begins with a rupture or erosion of plaque — an unstable and lipid-rich substance.

The rupture results in platelet adhesions, fibrin clot formation, and activation of thrombin.

A thrombus progresses and occludes blood flow. (An early thrombus doesn't necessarily block blood flow.) The effect is an imbalance in myocardial oxygen supply and demand. Depending on the degree of occlusion, ACS is defined as three types.

If the patient has unstable angina, a thrombus partially occludes a coronary vessel. This thrombus is full of platelets. The partially occluded vessel may have distal microthrombi that cause necrosis in some myocytes.

If smaller vessels infarct, the patient is at higher risk for MI, which may progress to a non-ST-segment elevation MI. Usually, only the inner-most layer of the heart is damaged.

ST-segment elevation MI results when reduced blood flow through one of the coronary arteries causes myocardial ischemia, injury, and necrosis. The damage extends through all myocardial layers.

ACS tissue destruction

The destruction of healthy cardiac tissue from myocardial ischemia varies with the severity of the ACS involved and the promptness of effective diagnosis and treatment.

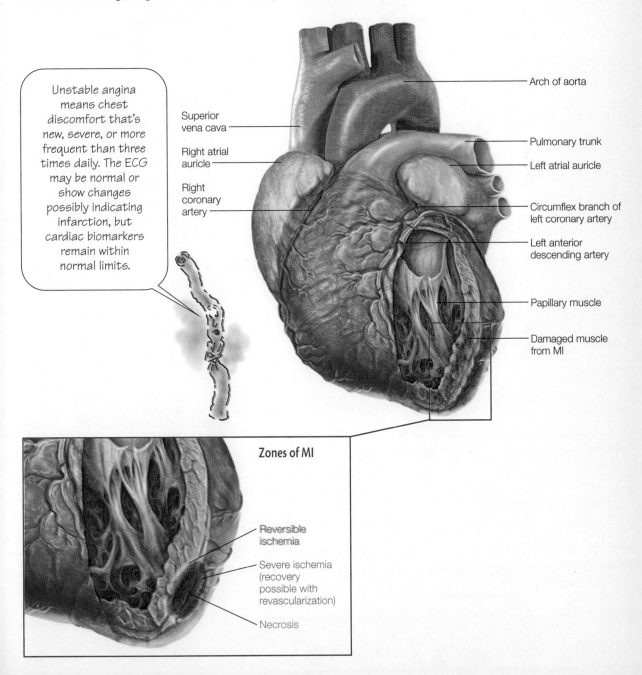

Unstable angina means chest discomfort that's new, severe, or more frequent than three times daily. The ECG may be normal or show changes possibly indicating infarction, but cardiac biomarkers remain within normal limits.

Superior vena cava

Right atrial auricle

Right coronary artery

Arch of aorta

Pulmonary trunk

Left atrial auricle

Circumflex branch of left coronary artery

Left anterior descending artery

Papillary muscle

Damaged muscle from MI

Zones of MI

Reversible ischemia

Severe ischemia (recovery possible with revascularization)

Necrosis

Comparing signs and symptoms: Unstable angina and MI

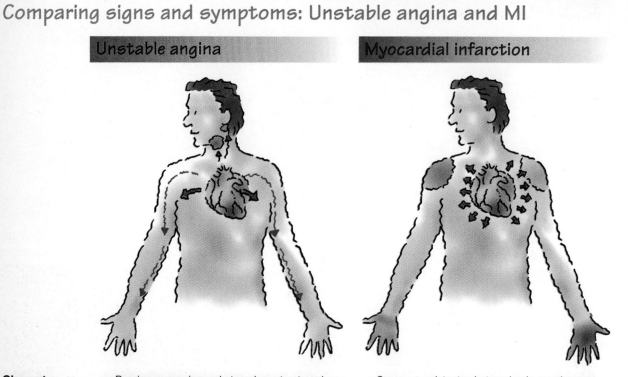

	Unstable angina	**Myocardial infarction**
Character, location, and radiation	■ Burning, squeezing, substernal or retrosternal pain spreading across chest; may radiate to inside of arm, neck, jaw, or shoulder blade	■ Severe, persistent substernal pain or pain over pericardium; may spread widely throughout chest and be accompanied by pain in shoulders and hands; may be described as crushing or squeezing
Duration of pain	■ 5 to 15 min	■ > 15 min
Precipitating events	■ Usually related to exertion, emotion, eating, cold	■ Occurs spontaneously ■ May be sequela to unstable angina
Relieving measures	■ Rest, nitroglycerin, oxygen	■ Morphine sulfate, successful reperfusion of blocked coronary artery
Associated symptoms	■ Shortness of breath ■ Dizziness ■ Nausea ■ Palpitations ■ Weakness ■ Cold sweat	■ Feeling of impending doom ■ Fatigue ■ Nausea and vomiting ■ Shortness of breath ■ Cool extremities ■ Perspiration ■ Anxiety
Associated signs	■ Hypotension or hypertension ■ Tachycardia or bradycardia	■ Hypotension or hypertension ■ Palpable precordial pulse ■ Muffled heart sounds ■ Arrhythmias
Cardiac biomarkers	■ Usually within normal range	■ Elevated

Atypical chest pain in women

Women with CAD may experience classic chest pain, which may occur without any relationship to activity or stress. However, they also commonly experience atypical chest pain, vague chest pain, or a lack of chest pain.

Location, location, location

Whereas men tend to complain of crushing pain in the center of the chest, women are more likely to experience arm or shoulder pain; jaw, neck, or throat pain; toothache; back pain; or pain under the breastbone or in the stomach.

Other signs and symptoms women may experience include nausea or dizziness; shortness of breath; unexplained anxiety, weakness, or fatigue; palpitations; cold sweat; or paleness.

> Any patient may experience atypical chest pain, but it's more common in women.

Rx

- Oxygen therapy
- Pain relief measures
- Reduced cardiac oxygen demand
- Prompt thrombolytic therapy, when possible, or angioplasty or bypass grafting
- Stabilization of heart rhythm, as needed

> Aloha!

memory board

The American Heart Association's acronym for saying goodbye to heart disease, **ALOHA,** can help you remember recommendations for your female patients who are at risk:
Assess your risk. Know important levels, such as cholesterol, weight, and blood pressure.
Lifestyle is the priority. Lifestyle changes, such as smoking cessation, exercise, and a healthy diet, can help prevent cardiovascular disease.
Other interventions may be necessary if lifestyle changes don't significantly reduce the risk of heart disease. Consult a physician.
High-risk cases are serious and need to be addressed immediately and consistently.
Avoid hormone therapy, antioxidant vitamin supplements, and aspirin therapy because these treatments may do more harm than good, especially in low-risk patients.

Vascular disorders

Vascular disorders can affect arteries, veins, or both. Arterial disorders include aneurysms, which result from weakening of the arterial wall, and arterial occlusive disease, which commonly results from atherosclerotic narrowing of the artery's lumen. Thrombophlebitis, a venous disorder, results from inflammation or occlusion of the affected vessel.

Aortic aneurysm

■ Localized outpouching or abnormal dilation in a weakened arterial wall of the aorta
■ When developing, lateral pressure increases, causing the vessel lumen to widen and blood flow to slow
■ May result in hemodynamic forces that cause pulsatile stresses on the weakened wall and press on the small vessels that supply nutrients to the arterial wall, causing the aorta to become bowed and tortuous.

Locations of aortic aneurysms

■ Syphilitic aneurysms are the common variety in the ascending aorta, which is usually spared by the atherosclerotic process.
■ Atherosclerotic aneurysms usually occur in the abdominal aorta or upper leg arteries.
■ Mycotic aneurysms occur anywhere that bacteria can deposit on vessel walls.
■ Dissecting-type aneurysms are most commonly seen in the descending or thoracic aorta.

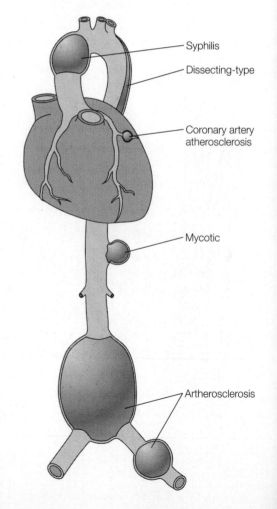

Syphilis

Dissecting-type

Coronary artery atherosclerosis

Mycotic

Artherosclerosis

Signs and symptoms

■ Possibly none when aneurysm is small (usually)
■ Pain, hypotension, and decreased peripheral circulation when aneurysm is large, leaking, or pressing on internal structures
■ Back pain, groin pain, and pulsating abdominal mass with rupture of abdominal aortic aneurysm

An aortic aneurysm may suddenly rupture or tear, possibly causing death. Rupture of an aortic aneurysm is a medical emergency requiring prompt treatment.

Types

Dissecting

A hemorrhagic separation in the aortic wall, usually within the medial layer

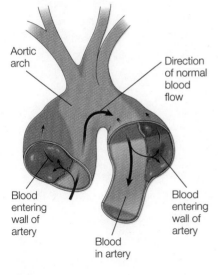

Aortic arch

Direction of normal blood flow

Blood entering wall of artery

Blood in artery

Blood entering wall of artery

Saccular

An outpouching of the arterial wall

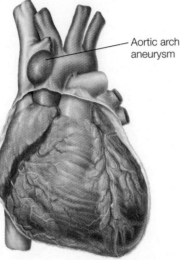

Aortic arch aneurysm

Fusiform

A fusiform aneurysm is a spindle-shaped enlargement encompassing the entire aortic circumference.

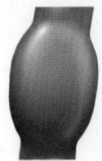

False

A false aneurysm occurs when the entire wall is injured, resulting in a break in all layers of the arterial wall. Blood leaks out, but is contained by the surrounding structures, creating a pulsatile hematoma.

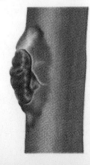

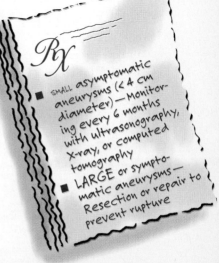

Rx

- SMALL asymptomatic aneurysms (< 4 cm diameter)—Monitoring every 6 months with ultrasonography, x-ray, or computed tomography
- LARGE or symptomatic aneurysms—Resection or repair to prevent rupture

Arterial occlusive disease

Arterial occlusive disease is a common complication of atherosclerosis. Obstruction or narrowing of the lumen of the aorta and its major branches causes an interruption of blood flow, usually to the legs and feet. It may affect the carotid, vertebral, subclavian, mesenteric, and celiac arteries and may be acute or chronic. Risk factors for arterial occlusive disease include smoking, aging, hypertension, hyperlipidemia, diabetes mellitus, and family history of vascular disorders, MI, or stroke. Men suffer from arterial occlusive disease more often than women.

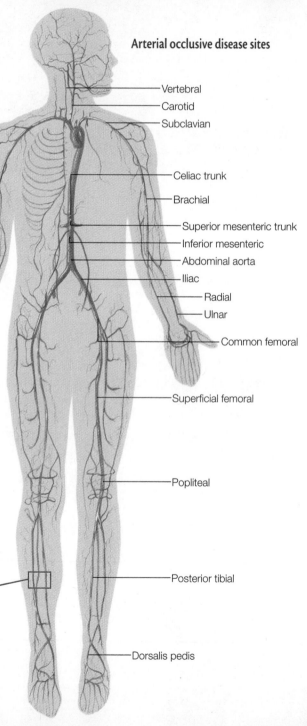

Arterial occlusive disease sites

- Vertebral
- Carotid
- Subclavian
- Celiac trunk
- Brachial
- Superior mesenteric trunk
- Inferior mesenteric
- Abdominal aorta
- Iliac
- Radial
- Ulnar
- Common femoral
- Superficial femoral
- Popliteal
- Posterior tibial
- Dorsalis pedis

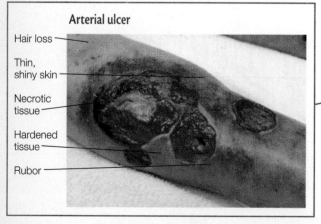

Arterial ulcer

- Hair loss
- Thin, shiny skin
- Necrotic tissue
- Hardened tissue
- Rubor

The five P's of acute occlusion

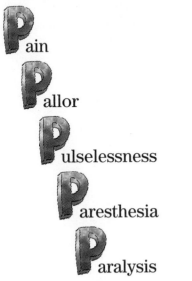

Pain

Pallor

Pulselessness

Paresthesia

Paralysis

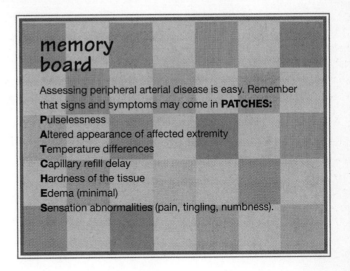

memory board

Assessing peripheral arterial disease is easy. Remember that signs and symptoms may come in **PATCHES**:

Pulselessness
Altered appearance of affected extremity
Temperature differences
Capillary refill delay
Hardness of the tissue
Edema (minimal)
Sensation abnormalities (pain, tingling, numbness).

Treating arterial occlusive disease

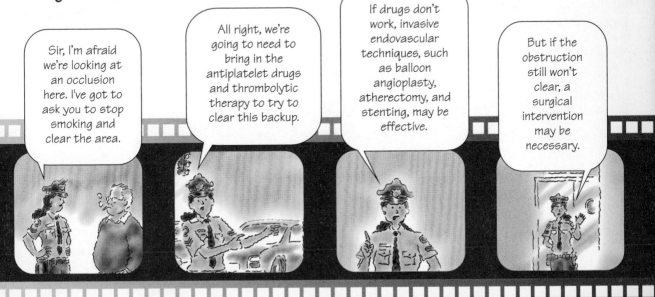

Sir, I'm afraid we're looking at an occlusion here. I've got to ask you to stop smoking and clear the area.

All right, we're going to need to bring in the antiplatelet drugs and thrombolytic therapy to try to clear this backup.

If drugs don't work, invasive endovascular techniques, such as balloon angioplasty, atherectomy, and stenting, may be effective.

But if the obstruction still won't clear, a surgical intervention may be necessary.

Thrombophlebitis

Thrombophlebitis is an acute condition characterized by inflammation and thrombus formation in the veins. Alteration in the epithelial lining causes platelet aggregation and fibrin entrapment of red blood cells (RBCs), white blood cells, and additional platelets. The thrombus initiates a chemical inflammatory process in the vessel epithelium that leads to fibrosis, which may occlude the vessel lumen or embolize.

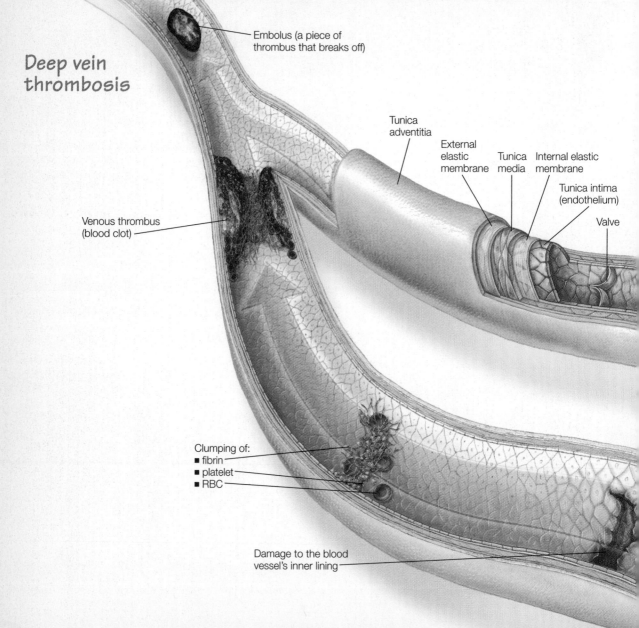

Embolus (a piece of thrombus that breaks off)

Deep vein thrombosis

Tunica adventitia

External elastic membrane

Tunica media

Internal elastic membrane

Tunica intima (endothelium)

Valve

Venous thrombus (blood clot)

Clumping of:
- fibrin
- platelet
- RBC

Damage to the blood vessel's inner lining

Superficial (subcutaneous) thrombophlebitis is usually self-limiting and rarely leads to pulmonary embolism.

Deep vein (intermuscular or intramuscular) thrombophlebitis can affect small veins as well as large veins, such as the vena cava and the femoral, iliac, and subclavian veins. Usually progressive, this disorder may lead to pulmonary embolism, a potentially fatal condition.

Signs and symptoms of superficial thrombophlebitis

Along the length of the affected vein:
- Heat
- Pain and tenderness
- Swelling
- Redness and induration

Signs and symptoms of DVT

- Fever and chills
- Malaise
- Severe pain
- Swelling of the extremity
- Cyanosis of the extremity distal to the blockage
- Positive Homans' sign

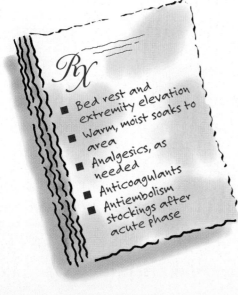

Rx
- Bed rest and extremity elevation
- Warm, moist soaks to area
- Analgesics, as needed
- Anticoagulants
- Antiembolism stockings after acute phase

A patient with a high risk of thrombophlebitis and pulmonary embolus who also has contraindications to anticoagulant therapy or a high risk of bleeding might undergo insertion of a vena caval umbrella or filter.

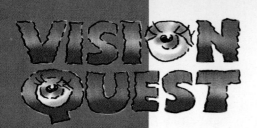

VISION QUEST

My word!

Use the clues to help you unscramble the names of three common cardiovascular disorders. Then use the circled letters to answer the question posed.

Question: Which form of hypertension, also known as primary hypertension, is the most common type?

1. Diffuse inflammation of the cardiac muscle

   mytacosridi

   _ _ _ _ _ ⃝ _ _ _ ⃝ _ ⃝

2. Ineffective myocardial pumping

   hrate irefaul

   _ ⃝ _ _ _   _ _ _ ⃝ _ _ _

3. Outpouching of the arterial wall

   actori mayersun

   _ _ _ _ ⃝ _   _ ⃝ ⃝ _ _ _ ⃝ _

   Answer: _ _ _ _ _ _ _ _ _ _

Matchmaker

Match the four aneurysms shown here with their names.

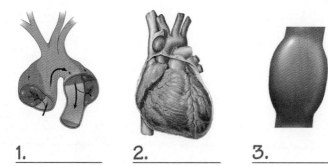 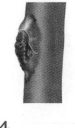

1. _____   2. _____   3. _____   4. _____

A. Saccular aortic
B. Fusiform
C. Dissecting aortic
D. False

172

7 Complications

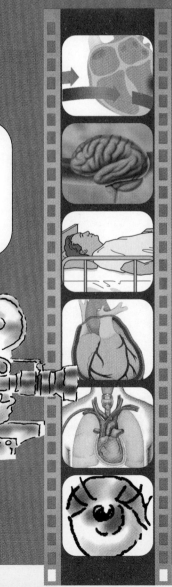

Cardiovascular care is complicated. You've got to keep your eye out for complications.

Cardiogenic shock

Cardiogenic shock is a commonly fatal complication of various acute and chronic disorders that can cause cardiac decompensation. It can result from any condition that causes significant left ventricular dysfunction and reduced cardiac output, with the most common cause being acute myocardial infarction (MI).

Cardiogenic shock is sometimes called *pump failure*. It causes cardiac output to diminish, which severely impairs tissue perfusion.

Signs and symptoms

- Cyanosis
- Metabolic acidosis
- Cool, clammy skin
- Weak, thready pulse

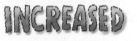

- Heart rate
- Respiration
- Pulmonary artery pressure (PAP) and pulmonary artery wedge pressure (PAWP)

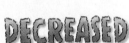

- Systolic pressure (< 80 mm Hg)
- Urine output (< 20 ml/hour)
- Pulse pressure
- Cardiac index
- Oxygen saturation

Cycle of decompensation

After an MI, even a slight reduction in cardiac output
and arterial pressure can initiate a cycle of cardiac
deterioration that results in cardiogenic shock.

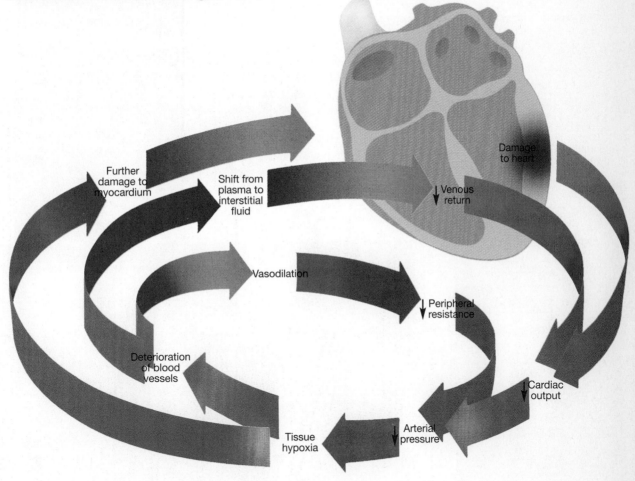

Further
damage to
myocardium

Shift from
plasma to
interstitial
fluid

Damage
to heart

↓ Venous
return

Vasodilation

↓ Peripheral
resistance

Deterioration
of blood
vessels

↓ Cardiac
output

Tissue
hypoxia

↓ Arterial
pressure

Hemodynamic abnormalities in cardiogenic shock

Parameter	Abnormal value
Right atrial pressure	6 to 10 mm Hg
Right ventricular pressure	40 to 50/6 to 15 mm Hg
PAP	50/25 to 30 mm Hg
PAWP	25 to 40 mm Hg
Cardiac output	<4 L/min
Cardiac index	<1.5 L/min/m^2

memory board

To help you recall the treatment protocol for cardiogenic shock, remember your ABCs (plus a D and an E).

Airway control with possible mechanical assistance

Breathing with high–flow rate oxygen therapy

Circulation monitoring and maintenance of large-bore I.V. lines

Drugs to increase cardiac output and stabilize hemodynamics

Emergency IABP or surgery

When drug therapy and IABP aren't enough, a ventricular assist device may provide the next line of defense.

Rx
- I.V. dopamine (Intropin), phenylephrine (Neo-Synephrine), or norepinephrine (Levophed)
- Inotropic agent, such as inamrinone (Amrinone) or dobutamine (Dobutrex)
- Intra-aortic balloon pump (IABP)
- Thrombolytic therapy or coronary artery revascularization
- Emergency surgery, if applicable

Hypovolemic shock

In hypovolemic shock, reduced intravascular volume causes circulatory dysfunction and inadequate tissue perfusion. It's commonly caused by acute blood loss—about 20% of total volume—that can result from:

■ GI bleeding, internal or external hemorrhage, or any condition that reduces circulating intravascular volume or levels of other body fluids
■ intestinal obstruction
■ peritonitis
■ acute pancreatitis
■ dehydration from excessive perspiration, severe diarrhea, protracted vomiting, diabetes insipidus, diuresis, or inadequate fluid intake.

Between a rock and a hard space

Third-space fluid shift can also cause hypovolemic shock. It can occur in the abdominal cavity (ascites), pleural cavity, or pericardial sac.

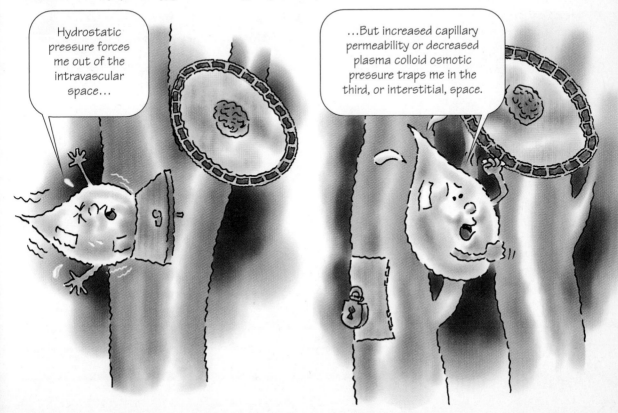

How hypovolemic shock occurs

The body initially tries to compensate for fluid loss; however, without prompt treatment, the body's compensatory mechanisms can't maintain circulation for long. Blood pressure falls dramatically and tissue perfusion decreases. The specific signs and symptoms that your patient exhibits will depend on the amount of fluid loss.

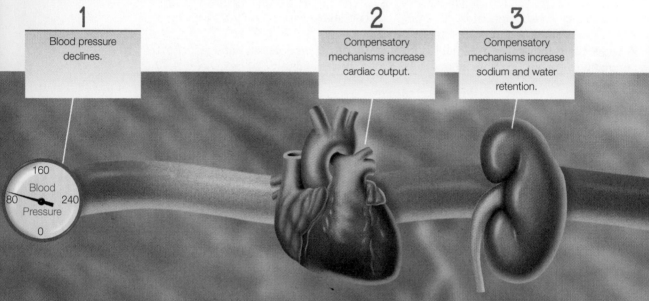

1 Blood pressure declines.

2 Compensatory mechanisms increase cardiac output.

3 Compensatory mechanisms increase sodium and water retention.

160
Blood
80   240
Pressure
0

Estimating fluid loss

Changes in your patient's blood pressure, pulse rate, urine output, mental status, and skin condition signal whether fluid loss is minimal, moderate, or severe.

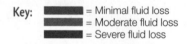

Key:
= Minimal fluid loss
= Moderate fluid loss
= Severe fluid loss

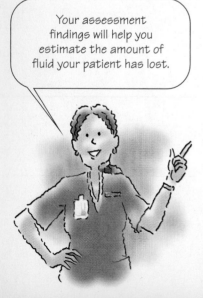

Your assessment findings will help you estimate the amount of fluid your patient has lost.

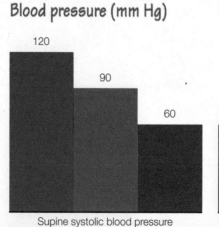

Blood pressure (mm Hg)

120

90

60

Supine systolic blood pressure

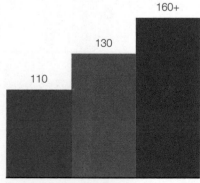

Pulse rate (beats/minute)

160+

130

110

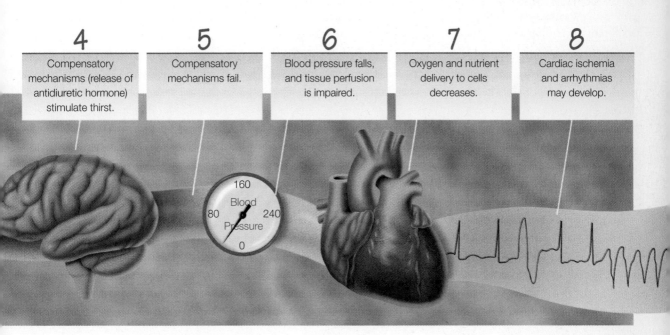

4 Compensatory mechanisms (release of antidiuretic hormone) stimulate thirst.

5 Compensatory mechanisms fail.

6 Blood pressure falls, and tissue perfusion is impaired.

7 Oxygen and nutrient delivery to cells decreases.

8 Cardiac ischemia and arrhythmias may develop.

160
Blood
80   240
Pressure
0

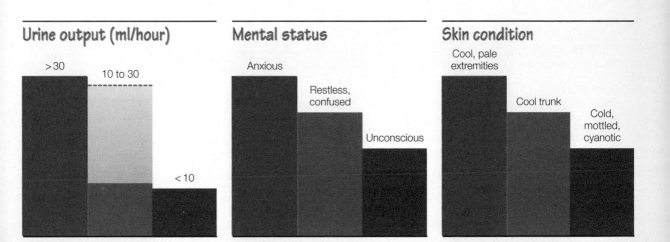

Urine output (ml/hour)

> 30

10 to 30

< 10

Mental status

Anxious

Restless, confused

Unconscious

Skin condition

Cool, pale extremities

Cool trunk

Cold, mottled, cyanotic

Signs and symptoms

■ Cyanosis
■ Metabolic acidosis
■ Cool, clammy skin
■ Weak, thready pulse

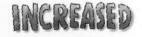

■ Heart rate
■ Respiration
■ Urine specific gravity
■ Potassium, creatinine, and blood urea nitrogen levels

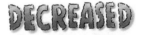

■ Sensorium
■ Pulse pressure
■ Urine output (less than 25 ml/hour)
■ Blood pressure
■ Central venous pressure (CVP), PAP, and PAWP
■ Hemoglobin level
■ Hematocrit

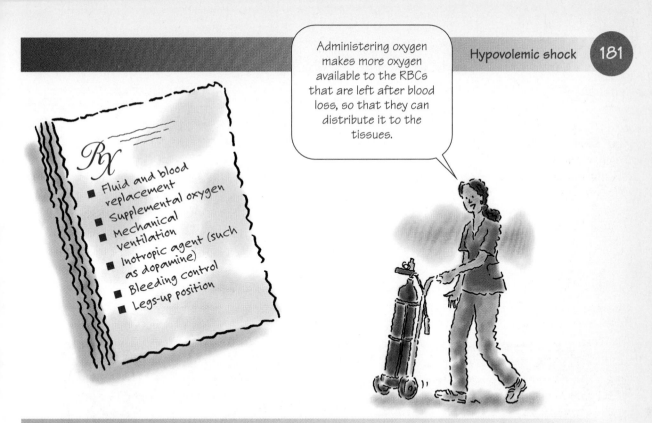

Administering oxygen makes more oxygen available to the RBCs that are left after blood loss, so that they can distribute it to the tissues.

Rx

- Fluid and blood replacement
- Supplemental oxygen
- Mechanical ventilation
- Inotropic agent (such as dopamine)
- Bleeding control
- Legs-up position

Positioning for shock

For years, patients in hypovolemic shock were placed in Trendelenburg's position. However, research now shows that only the legs should be significantly elevated to avoid affecting gas exchange in the lungs.

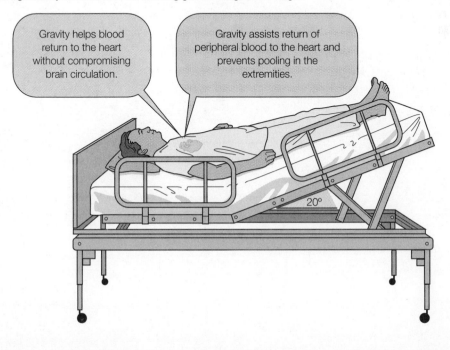

Gravity helps blood return to the heart without compromising brain circulation.

Gravity assists return of peripheral blood to the heart and prevents pooling in the extremities.

20°

Cardiac tamponade

Cardiac tamponade is an unchecked increase in pressure in the pericardial sac. It usually results from blood or fluid that accumulates in the sac and compresses the heart. This compression obstructs blood flow to the ventricles and reduces the amount of blood pumped out of the heart with each contraction. Possible causes include Dressler's syndrome, MI, pericarditis, malignant effusions, or a reaction to certain drugs, such as procainamide (Pronestyl) or hydralazine (Apresoline).

MI and cardiac tamponade

A ruptured MI causes a massive accumulation of blood in the pericardial cavity. The result is cardiac tamponade.

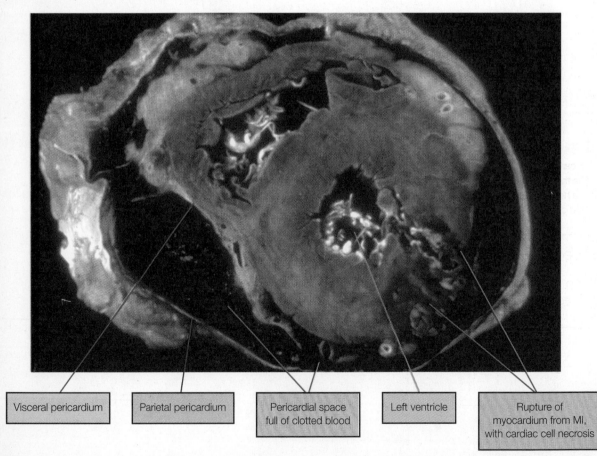

| Visceral pericardium | Parietal pericardium | Pericardial space full of clotted blood | Left ventricle | Rupture of myocardium from MI, with cardiac cell necrosis |

Understanding cardiac tamponade

Normal heart and pericardium

The pericardial space normally contains 10 to 30 ml of pericardial fluid, which lubricates the layers of the heart and reduces friction when the heart contracts.

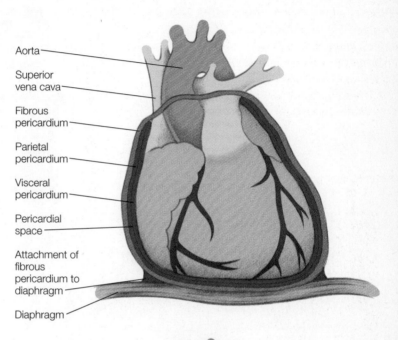

Aorta

Superior vena cava

Fibrous pericardium

Parietal pericardium

Visceral pericardium

Pericardial space

Attachment of fibrous pericardium to diaphragm

Diaphragm

Cardiac tamponade

In cardiac tamponade, blood or fluid fills the pericardial space, compressing the heart, decreasing cardiac output, and obstructing venous return.

Even a small amount of fluid — 50 to 100 ml — can be fatal if it accumulates rapidly.

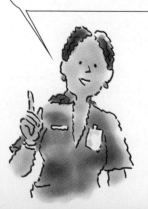

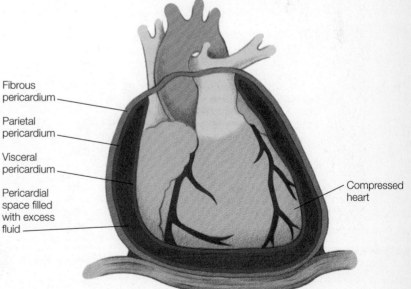

Fibrous pericardium

Parietal pericardium

Visceral pericardium

Pericardial space filled with excess fluid

Compressed heart

Signs and symptoms

The three classic signs of cardiac tamponade are:
- elevated CVP with jugular vein distention
- muffled heart sounds
- pulsus paradoxus (inspiratory drop in systemic blood pressure greater than 15 mm Hg).

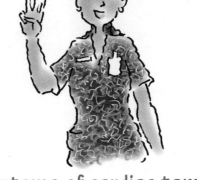

Cardiac tamponade has three classic features known as Beck's triad.

Understanding signs and symptoms of cardiac tamponade

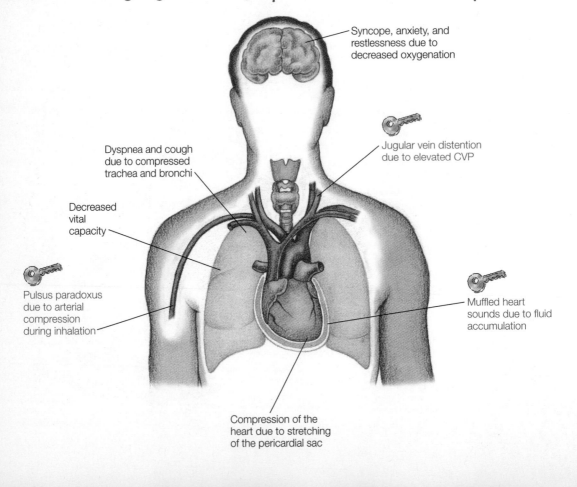

Syncope, anxiety, and restlessness due to decreased oxygenation

Jugular vein distention due to elevated CVP

Dyspnea and cough due to compressed trachea and bronchi

Decreased vital capacity

Pulsus paradoxus due to arterial compression during inhalation

Muffled heart sounds due to fluid accumulation

Compression of the heart due to stretching of the pericardial sac

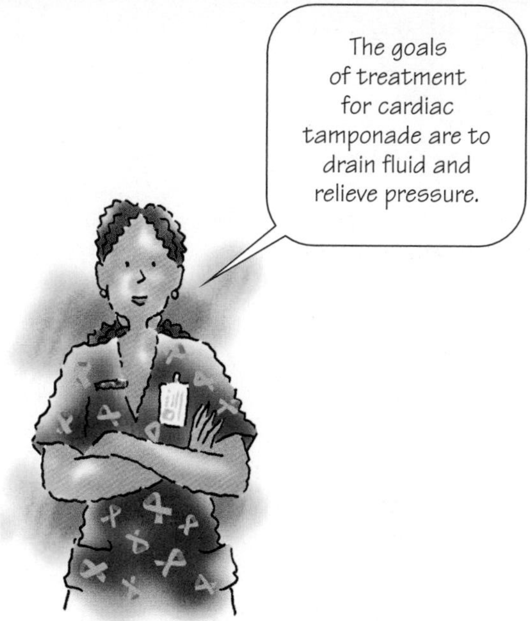

The goals of treatment for cardiac tamponade are to drain fluid and relieve pressure.

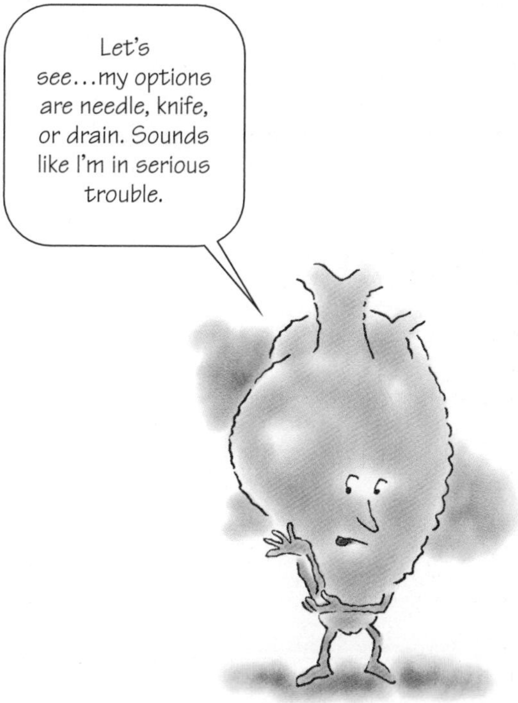

Let's see…my options are needle, knife, or drain. Sounds like I'm in serious trouble.

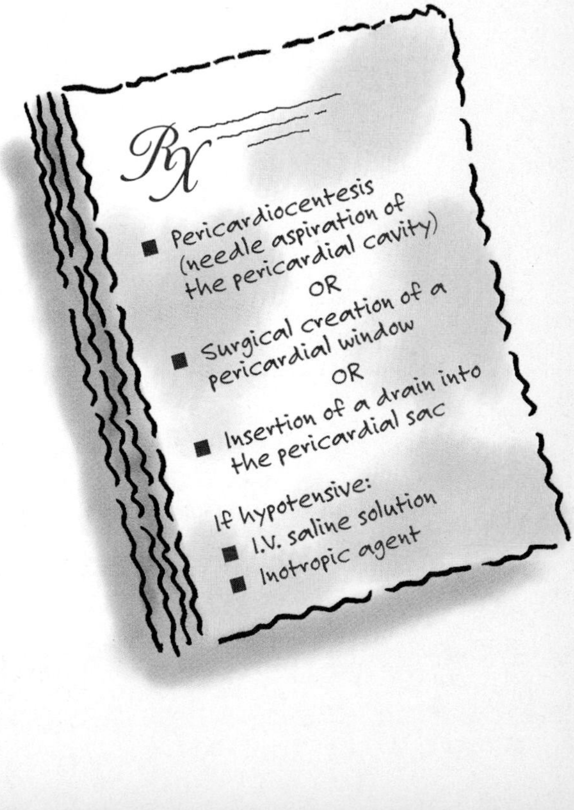

Rx

- Pericardiocentesis (needle aspiration of the pericardial cavity)
  OR
- Surgical creation of a pericardial window
  OR
- Insertion of a drain into the pericardial sac

If hypotensive:
- I.V. saline solution
- Inotropic agent

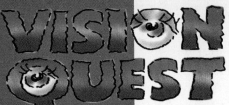

Rebus riddle

Sound out each group of symbols and letters to reveal a fact about a cardiovascular complication.

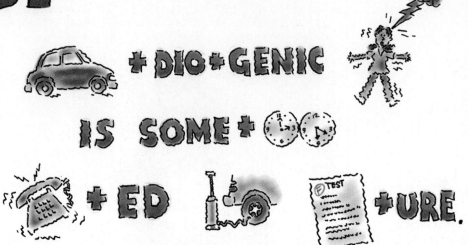

My word!

Unscramble the names of four terms related to cardiac tamponade. Then use the circled letters to answer the question posed.

Question: What name is given to the three classic signs of cardiac tamponade?

1. carriedpail capes

_ _ _ _ _ _ ◯ _ _ ◯ _ _ ◯ _ _ _ _ _

2. mrspoonsice

◯ _ _ _ ◯ _ _ _ _

3. lobdo tunicacoalum

◯ _ _ _ _ _ _ _ _ _ _ _ ◯ _ _

4. needchuck canesire

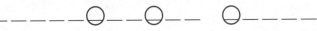
_ _ _ _ _ _ _ ◯ ◯ _ _ _ _ ◯ _ _

Answer: _ _ _ _ _ ' _ _ _ _ _ _

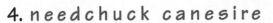
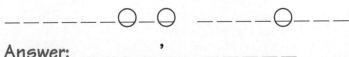
186

8 Treatments

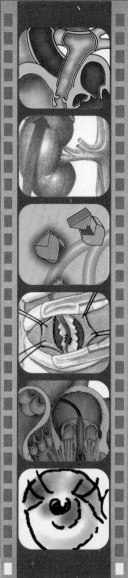

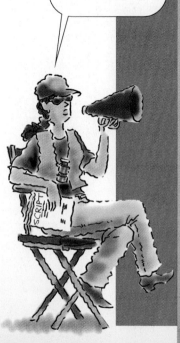

Some movie stars require careful treatment. Patients require careful treatment, too!

Drug therapy

■ Antiarrhythmics

Antiarrhythmics are used to treat disturbances in normal heart rhythm and are grouped in one of four classes.

> As far as class I antiarrhythmics go, I'm a class act. But I'm also in a class of my own.

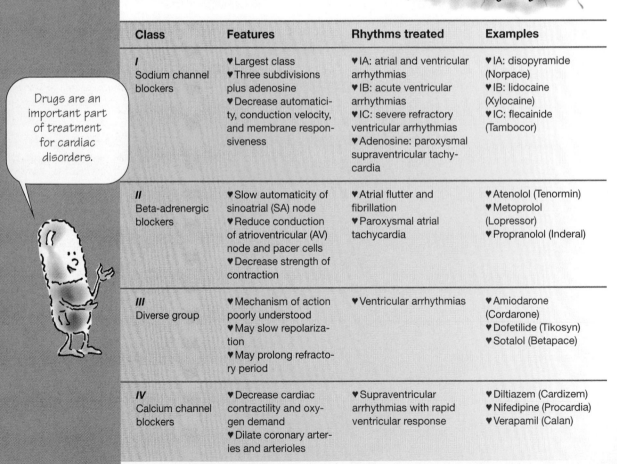

> Drugs are an important part of treatment for cardiac disorders.

Class	Features	Rhythms treated	Examples
I Sodium channel blockers	♥ Largest class ♥ Three subdivisions plus adenosine ♥ Decrease automaticity, conduction velocity, and membrane responsiveness	♥ IA: atrial and ventricular arrhythmias ♥ IB: acute ventricular arrhythmias ♥ IC: severe refractory ventricular arrhythmias ♥ Adenosine: paroxysmal supraventricular tachycardia	♥ IA: disopyramide (Norpace) ♥ IB: lidocaine (Xylocaine) ♥ IC: flecainide (Tambocor)
II Beta-adrenergic blockers	♥ Slow automaticity of sinoatrial (SA) node ♥ Reduce conduction of atrioventricular (AV) node and pacer cells ♥ Decrease strength of contraction	♥ Atrial flutter and fibrillation ♥ Paroxysmal atrial tachycardia	♥ Atenolol (Tenormin) ♥ Metoprolol (Lopressor) ♥ Propranolol (Inderal)
III Diverse group	♥ Mechanism of action poorly understood ♥ May slow repolarization ♥ May prolong refractory period	♥ Ventricular arrhythmias	♥ Amiodarone (Cordarone) ♥ Dofetilide (Tikosyn) ♥ Sotalol (Betapace)
IV Calcium channel blockers	♥ Decrease cardiac contractility and oxygen demand ♥ Dilate coronary arteries and arterioles	♥ Supraventricular arrhythmias with rapid ventricular response	♥ Diltiazem (Cardizem) ♥ Nifedipine (Procardia) ♥ Verapamil (Calan)

Inotropic drugs

Inotropics increase the force of the heart's contractions. There are two types:
- digoxin (Lanoxin), which slows the heart rate and electrical impulse conduction through the SA and AV nodes
- phosphodiesterase (PDE) inhibitors, which provide short-term management of heart failure or long-term management in patients awaiting heart transplant surgery. Two examples of PDE inhibitors are inamrinone and milrinone (Primacor).

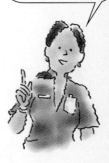

PDE inhibitors should be administered only via I.V.

Antianginals

Antianginals relieve chest pain by reducing myocardial oxygen demand, increasing the supply of oxygen to the heart, or both. There are three main types:
- nitrates (used primarily to treat acute angina)
- beta-adrenergic blockers (prescribed for long-term prevention of angina)
- calcium channel blockers (used when other drugs fail to prevent angina).

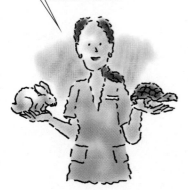

Nitrates can be quick or slow acting. It all depends on the delivery route and the drug.

How antianginal drugs work

When the coronary arteries can't supply enough oxygen to the myocardium, angina occurs. This forces the heart to work harder, increasing heart rate, preload, afterload, and the force of myocardial contractility. Antianginal drugs relieve angina by decreasing one or more of these four factors.

Afterload
- Calcium channel blockers
- Nitrates

Heart rate
- Beta-adrenergic blockers
- Calcium channel blockers

Preload
- Nitrates

Contractility
- Beta-adrenergic blockers
- Calcium channel blockers

Antihypertensives

Treatment for hypertension begins with modifying diet, encouraging exercise and, if indicated, counseling about weight loss. If these measures aren't enough, drugs can help.

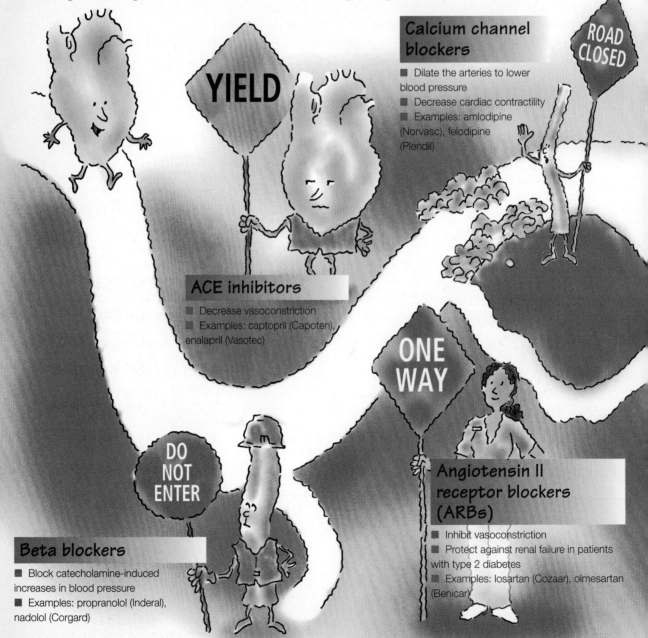

Calcium channel blockers
- Dilate the arteries to lower blood pressure
- Decrease cardiac contractility
- Examples: amlodipine (Norvasc), felodipine (Plendil)

ACE inhibitors
- Decrease vasoconstriction
- Examples: captopril (Capoten), enalapril (Vasotec)

Angiotensin II receptor blockers (ARBs)
- Inhibit vasoconstriction
- Protect against renal failure in patients with type 2 diabetes
- Examples: losartan (Cozaar), olmesartan (Benicar)

Beta blockers
- Block catecholamine-induced increases in blood pressure
- Examples: propranolol (Inderal), nadolol (Corgard)

Sympatholytics

■ Decrease peripheral vascular resistance by inhibiting the sympathetic nervous system
■ Examples: clonidine (Catapres), doxazosin (Cardura), carvedilol (Coreg)

SPEED
120 / 70
LIMIT

SLIPPERY WHEN WET

DETOUR

RESUME SPEED

Diuretics

■ Help kidneys excrete water and electrolytes, which lowers blood pressure
■ Thiazide example: hydrochlorothiazide (HydroDIURIL)
■ Loop example: furosemide (Lasix)
■ Potassium-sparing example: spironolactone (Aldactone)

Selective aldosterone receptor antagonists

■ Used as a second-line treatment when other drugs fail
■ Only example: eplerenone (Inspra)

Vasodilators

■ Relax arteries, veins, or both
■ Oral example: hydralazine (Apresoline)

For hypertensive crisis

■ Examples: I.V. nitroprusside (Nitropress), diazoxide (Hyperstat IV)

Treating hypertension

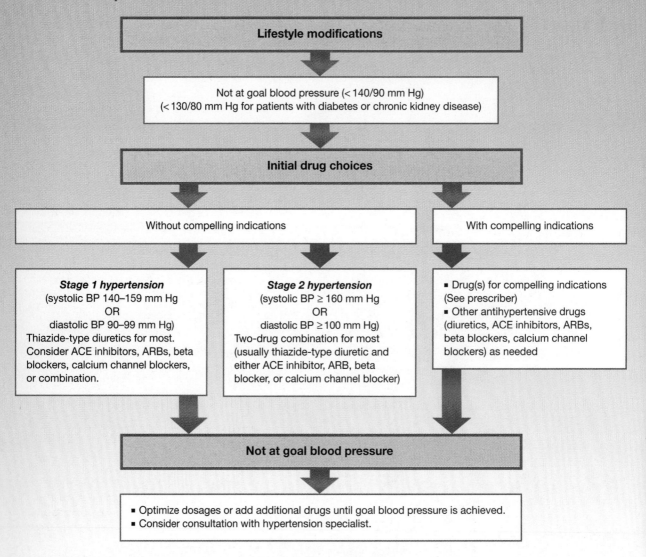

Lifestyle modifications

↓

Not at goal blood pressure (< 140/90 mm Hg)
(< 130/80 mm Hg for patients with diabetes or chronic kidney disease)

↓

Initial drug choices

Without compelling indications | **With compelling indications**

Stage 1 hypertension
(systolic BP 140–159 mm Hg
OR
diastolic BP 90–99 mm Hg)
Thiazide-type diuretics for most.
Consider ACE inhibitors, ARBs, beta blockers, calcium channel blockers, or combination.

Stage 2 hypertension
(systolic BP ≥ 160 mm Hg
OR
diastolic BP ≥ 100 mm Hg)
Two-drug combination for most (usually thiazide-type diuretic and either ACE inhibitor, ARB, beta blocker, or calcium channel blocker)

- Drug(s) for compelling indications (See prescriber)
- Other antihypertensive drugs (diuretics, ACE inhibitors, ARBs, beta blockers, calcium channel blockers) as needed

↓

Not at goal blood pressure

↓

- Optimize dosages or add additional drugs until goal blood pressure is achieved.
- Consider consultation with hypertension specialist.

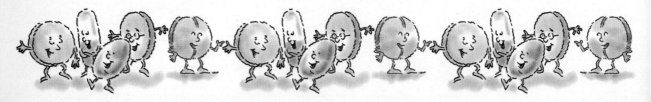

Antihypertensives and the RAAS

The renin-angiotensin-aldosterone system (RAAS) regulates the body's sodium and water levels and blood pressure.

1 Juxtaglomerular cells near the glomeruli in each kidney secrete the enzyme renin into the blood.

2 Renin circulates throughout the body and converts angiotensinogen, made in the liver, to angiotensin I.

3 In the lungs, angiotensin I is converted by hydrolysis to angiotensin II.

4 Angiotensin II acts on the adrenal cortex to stimulate production of the hormone aldosterone. Aldosterone acts on the juxtaglomerular cells to increase sodium and water retention and to stimulate or depress further renin secretion, completing the feedback system that automatically readjusts homeostasis.

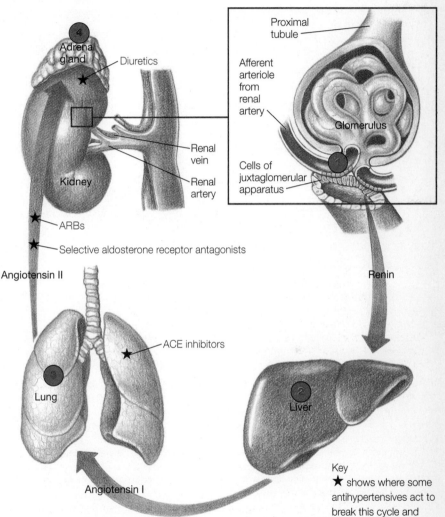

If your patient is taking an antihypertensive drug, watch for these signs and symptoms that may signal an adverse reaction.

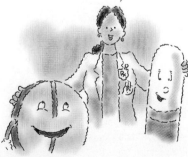

Key
★ shows where some antihypertensives act to break this cycle and lower blood pressure.

Adverse reactions of antihypertensive drugs

All

- Headache
- Fatigue
- Angioedema
- GI reactions
- Electrolyte imbalance (specific to drug used)

ACE inhibitors

- Altered renal function when used with non-steroidal anti-inflammatory drugs
- Dry, nonproductive, persistent cough

ARBs

- Transient elevations of blood urea nitrogen and serum creatinine levels
- Cough
- Tickling in throat

Antilipemics

Antilipemics lower cholesterol, triglyceride, and phospholipid levels. They're used in combination with lifestyle changes to decrease the risk of coronary artery disease (CAD).

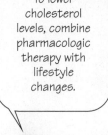

To lower cholesterol levels, combine pharmacologic therapy with lifestyle changes.

Cholesterol absorption inhibitors
- Lower total cholesterol levels
- Example: ezetimibe (Zetia)

Nicotinic acid (niacin)
- Water-soluble vitamin
- Lowers triglyceride levels
- Increases high-density lipoprotein (HDL) levels

Bile-sequestering drugs
- Remove excess bile acids from fat deposits
- Lower low-density lipoprotein (LDL) levels
- Example: cholestyramine (Questran)

Fibric-acid derivatives
- Lower triglyceride levels
- Minimally increase HDL levels
- Examples: fenofibrate (Tricor), gemfibrozil (Lopid)

HMG-CoA reductase inhibitors
- Also known as *statins*
- Lower total cholesterol and LDL levels
- Minimally increase HDL levels
- Examples: atorvastatin (Lipitor), simvastatin (Zocor)

Anticoagulants

Anticoagulants reduce the blood's ability to clot. They're prescribed for mitral insufficiency or atrial fibrillation or to dissolve clots that block an artery.

Category	Features	Examples
Heparins	♥Used in patients with unstable angina, MI, and deep vein thrombosis (DVT) ♥Act immediately when given I.V. ♥Available in regular and low-molecular-weight forms	♥Heparin (Liquaemin) *Low-molecular-weight* ♥Dalteparin (Fragmin) ♥Enoxaparin (Lovenox)
Coumarin derivative	♥Antagonizes production of vitamin K–dependent clotting factors ♥Prevents DVT ♥Used in patients who have undergone prosthetic heart valve surgery and those with diseased valves ♥Takes days to reach effect ♥Available only in oral form	♥Warfarin (Coumadin)
Antiplatelet drugs	♥Prevent thromboembolism	♥Aspirin ♥Clopidogrel (Plavix) ♥Dipyridamole (Persantine) ♥Sulfinpyrazone (Anturane) ♥Ticlopidine (Ticlid)
Direct thrombin inhibitors	♥Treat heparin-induced thrombocytopenia ♥Used when heparin can't be ♥Prophylactically used before angioplasty and stent placement ♥Available I.V.	♥Argatroban ♥Bivalirudin (Angiomax) ♥Lepirudin (Refludan)
Activated factor X inhibitor	♥Prevents DVT after total hip or knee replacement surgery or postoperatively with hip fractures	♥Fondaparinux (Arixtra)

■ Thrombolytics

Thrombolytics can dissolve a preexisting clot or thrombus in acute MI or ischemic stroke or peripheral artery occlusion. They also can dissolve thrombi and reestablish blood flow in arteriovenous cannulas and I.V. catheters. In an acute or emergency situation, they must be administered within 3 to 6 hours after the onset of symptoms. Thrombolytics include alteplase (Activase), reteplase (Retavase), streptokinase (Streptase), and urokinase (Abbokinase).

How thrombolytics help restore circulation

When a thrombus forms in an artery, it obstructs the blood supply, causing ischemia and necrosis. Thrombolytics can dissolve thrombi in the coronary and pulmonary arteries, restoring the blood supply to the area beyond the blockage.

Obstructed artery

A thrombus blocks blood flow through the artery, causing distal ischemia.

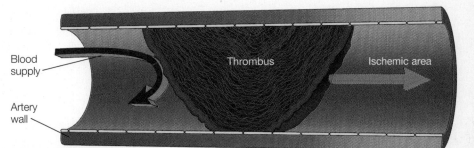

Inside the thrombus

The thrombolytic enters the thrombus and binds to the fibrin-plasminogen complex, converting inactive plasminogen into active plasmin. Active plasmin digests fibrin, dissolving the thrombus. As the thrombus dissolves, blood flow resumes.

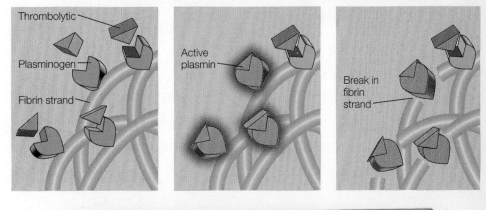

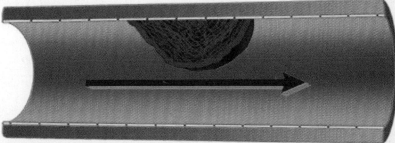

Treatments for CAD

Coronary artery bypass graft surgery

Coronary artery bypass graft (CABG) surgery relieves the symptoms of CAD and decreases risk of future heart attack or heart failure. Watch patients who have had CABG surgery for such complications as severe hypotension, decreased cardiac output, and cardiogenic shock.

> CABG circumvents an occluded coronary artery by using a segment of the saphenous vein, radial artery, or internal mammary artery to restore blood flow to the heart.

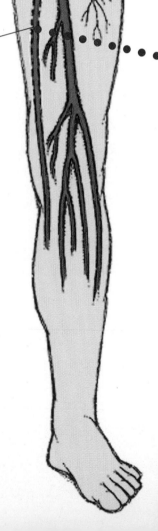

Greater saphenous vein

Donor vein

Internal
mammary
artery graft

Greater
saphenous
vein graft

photo op

Performing CABG surgery

CABG surgery is performed either "on pump" (the traditional method) or "off pump" (also called the "beating heart method" or OPCAB). A technician monitors the heart-lung machine (cardiopulmonary bypass pump), shown below.

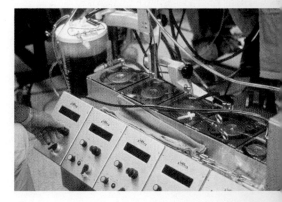

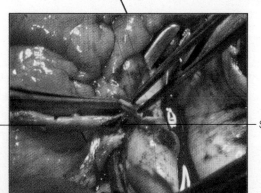

Donor
vein

Sutures

The road to recovery

Here are the landmarks that you'll want to look for on your patient's postoperative CABG road to recovery.

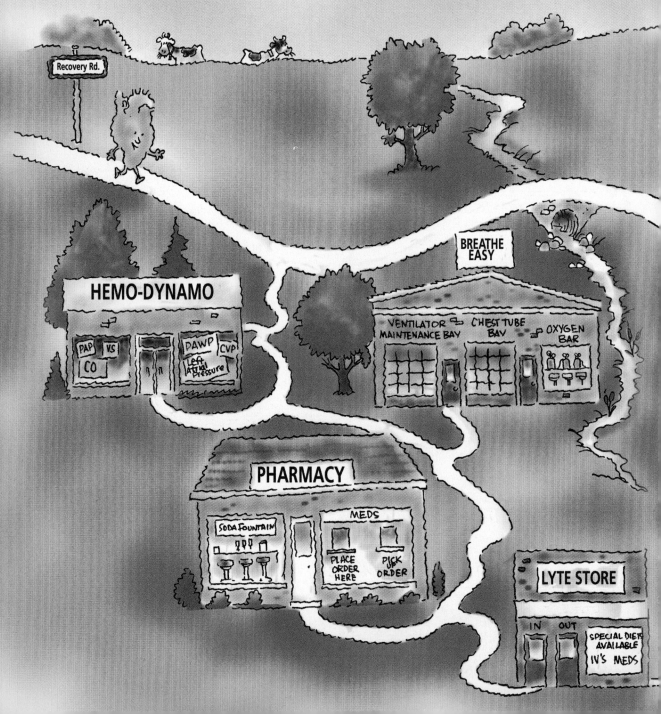

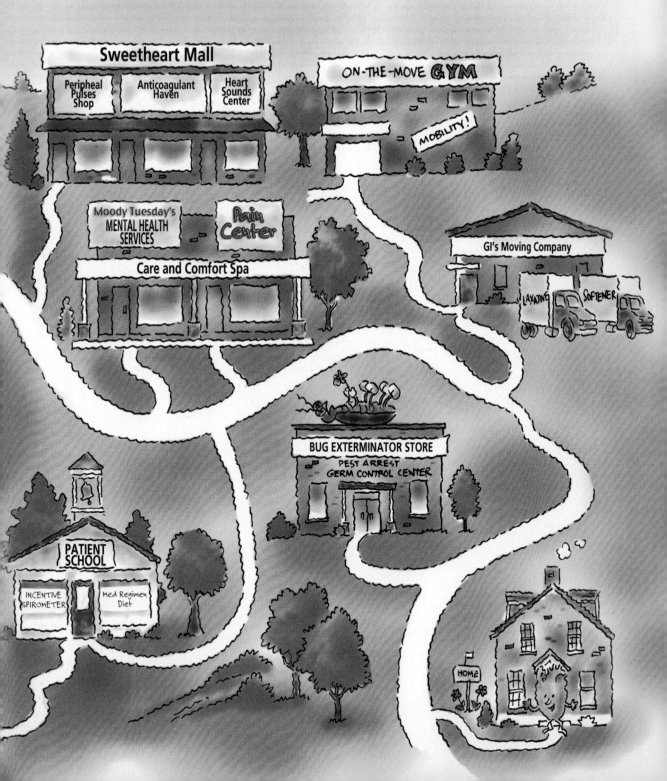

Minimally invasive direct coronary artery bypass

Minimally invasive direct coronary artery bypass (MIDCAB) is performed on a beating heart through a small thoracotomy incision. The patient receives only right lung ventilation and drugs to slow the heart rate and reduce heart movement during surgery. Because the procedure is minimally invasive, it results in shorter hospital stays, fewer post-operative complications, earlier extubation, reduced cost, smaller incisions, and an earlier return to work.

The MIDCAB procedure

MIDCAB is performed through a short incision in the left chest cavity. The internal mammary artery is sewn to the left anterior descending artery in the front of the heart, as shown here.

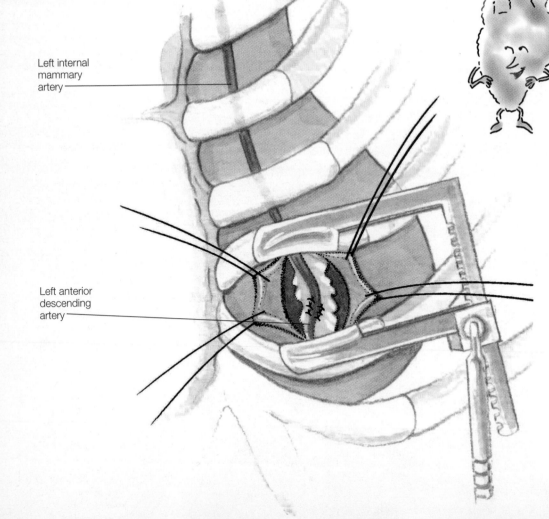

Left internal
mammary
artery

Left anterior
descending
artery

Comparing types of CABG

Features	On-pump CABG	OPCAB	MIDCAB
Access site	♥ Breastbone severed for heart access	♥ Breastbone severed for heart access	♥ Incision made between ribs for anterior heart access, no bones cut
Indications	♥ Suitable for multivessel disease, any coronary artery	♥ Suitable for multivessel disease, any coronary artery	♥ Only used for one-vessel diseases in anterior portions of heart, such as left anterior descending artery, or some portions of the right coronary and circumflex arteries
Graft types	♥ Combination of artery and vein grafts	♥ Combination of artery and vein grafts	♥ Arterial grafts (better long-term results)
Complications	♥ Highest risk of postoperative complications	♥ Reduced blood usage, fewer rhythm problems, less kidney dysfunction than on-pump CABG	♥ Reduced blood usage, fewest complications, fastest recovery
Intubation	♥ Up to 24 hours	♥ Up to 24 hours	♥ Usually for 2 to 4 hours
Incisions	♥ Leg incisions for vein grafting, possibly arm incision for radial artery grafting	♥ Leg incisions for vein grafting, possibly arm incision for radial artery grafting	♥ No leg incisions, possibly arm incision for radial artery grafting
Heart and lung function	♥ Heart and lung circulation bypassed mechanically, affecting blood cells	♥ Drugs and special equipment used to slow heart and immobilize it; cardiopulmonary and systemic circulation still function	♥ Drugs used to slow heart; cardiopulmonary and systemic circulation still function

Of the three types of CABG surgery, MIDCAB is the least invasive and has the fewest complications.

Percutaneous transluminal coronary angioplasty

Percutaneous transluminal coronary angioplasty (PTCA), also called *angioplasty*, is a nonsurgical alternative to CABG. Performed in the cardiac catheterization laboratory under local anesthesia, it involves the use of a balloon-tipped catheter to dilate the blocked coronary artery. In most cases, patients recuperate quickly, usually walking the same day and returning to work in 2 weeks.

PTCA works best when lesions are readily accessible, noncalcified, less than 10 mm, concentric, discrete, and smoothly tapered. Possible complications include acute vessel closure and late restenosis.

Understanding PTCA

In PTCA, a guide catheter is threaded into the coronary artery. Then a balloon-tipped catheter is inserted through the occlusion and inflated and deflated to flatten the plaque until the vessel is opened.

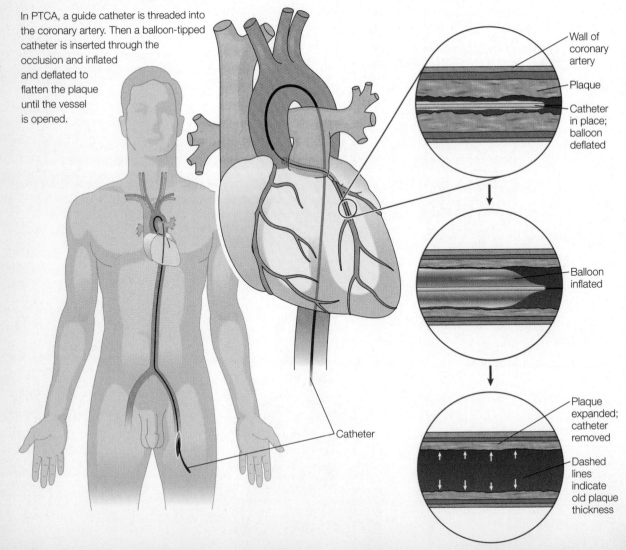

Wall of coronary artery

Plaque

Catheter in place; balloon deflated

Catheter

Balloon inflated

Plaque expanded; catheter removed

Dashed lines indicate old plaque thickness

Intravascular stents

An intravascular stent may be used to hold the walls of a vessel open. Some stents are coated with a drug that's slowly released to inhibit further aggregation of fibrin or clots.

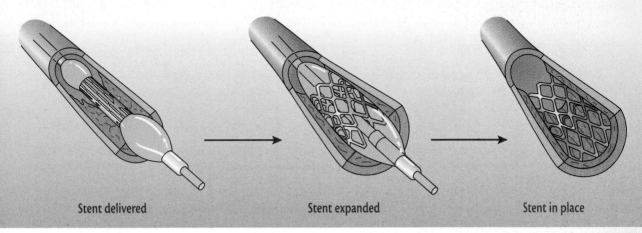

| Stent delivered | Stent expanded | Stent in place |

Atherectomy

Atherectomy is the use of a small, rotating knife to remove fatty deposits from blocked coronary arteries. The catheter is advanced to the arterial obstruction, the knife is positioned precisely on the fatty deposit, and then the fatty deposit is shaved off the artery wall.

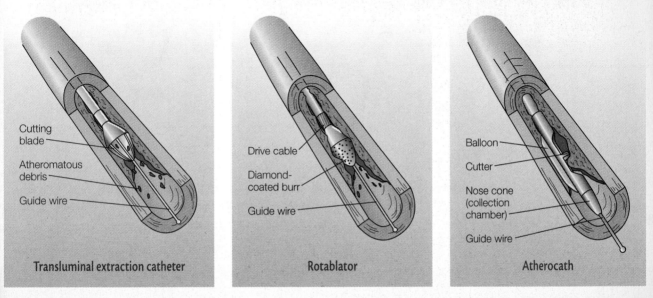

Cutting blade
Atheromatous debris
Guide wire

Transluminal extraction catheter

Drive cable
Diamond-coated burr
Guide wire

Rotablator

Balloon
Cutter
Nose cone (collection chamber)
Guide wire

Atherocath

IABP counterpulsation

Intra-aortic balloon pump (IABP) counterpulsation temporarily reduces left ventricular workload and improves coronary perfusion. It's used to treat cardiogenic shock caused by acute MI, septic shock, intractable angina before surgery, intractable ventricular arrhythmias, ventricular septal or papillary muscle ruptures, and pump failure.

Understanding an IABP

An IABP consists of a polyurethane balloon attached to an external pump console by means of a large-lumen catheter. It's inserted percutaneously through the femoral artery and positioned in the descending aorta, just distal to the left subclavian artery and above the renal arteries.

Push...

This external pump works in precise counterpoint to the left ventricle, inflating the balloon with helium early in diastole and deflating it just before systole. As the balloon inflates, it forces blood toward the aortic valve, thereby raising pressure in the aortic root and augmenting diastolic pressure to improve coronary perfusion. It also improves peripheral circulation by forcing blood through the brachiocephalic, common carotid, and subclavian arteries arising from the aortic trunk.

...and pull

The balloon deflates rapidly at the end of diastole, creating a vacuum in the aorta. This reduces aortic volume and pressure, thereby decreasing the resistance to left ventricular ejection (afterload). This decreased workload, in turn, reduces the heart's oxygen requirements and, combined with the improved myocardial perfusion, helps prevent or diminish myocardial ischemia.

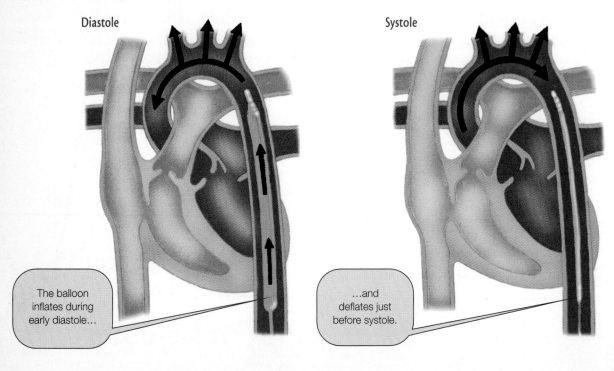

Diastole

The balloon inflates during early diastole...

Systole

...and deflates just before systole.

Timing IABP counterpulsation

IABP counterpulsation is synchronized with either the electrocardiogram or the arterial waveform. Ideally, balloon inflation should begin when the aortic valve closes — at the dicrotic notch on the arterial waveform. Deflation should occur just before systole.

When the time is right

Timing is crucial. Early inflation can damage the aortic valve by forcing it closed, whereas late inflation permits most of the blood emerging from the ventricle to flow past the balloon, reducing pump effectiveness.

Late deflation may cause cardiac arrest because it increases the resistance to left ventricle pumping.

At the peak

IABP counterpulsation boosts peak diastolic pressure and lowers peak systolic and end-diastolic pressures.

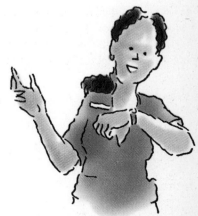

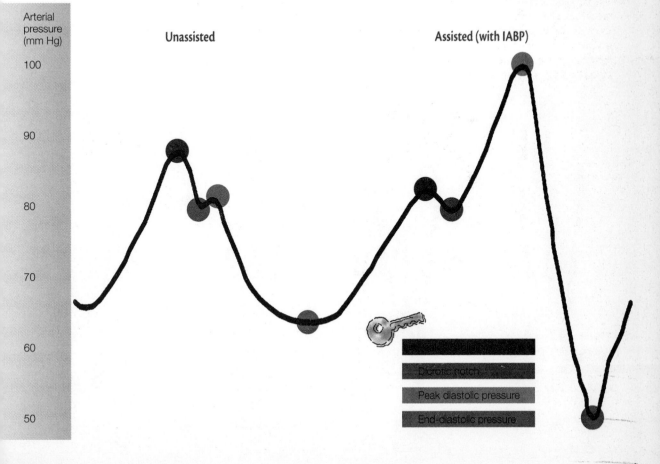

Arterial pressure (mm Hg)

Unassisted

Assisted (with IABP)

100

90

80

70

60

50

Peak systolic pressure

Dicrotic notch

Peak diastolic pressure

End-diastolic pressure

Enhanced external counterpulsation

Enhanced external counterpulsation (EECP) provides pain relief for patients who suffer from recurrent stable angina when standard treatments fail. It's a noninvasive technique that increases oxygen-rich blood flow to the heart and reduces the heart's workload. EECP can reduce angina pain, improve exercise tolerance, and stimulate collateral circulation.

EECP treatment

In EECP, three pneumatic cuffs are wrapped around the patient's calves, thighs, and lower buttocks. These cuffs sequentially inflate and gently compress blood vessels in the legs, forcing blood back to the heart.

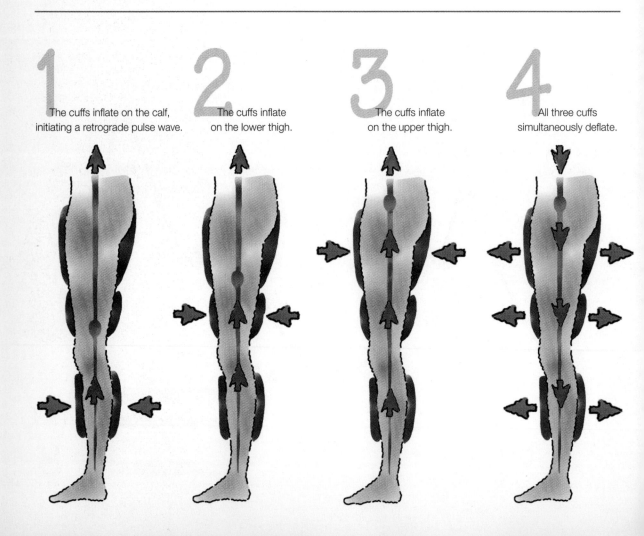

1 The cuffs inflate on the calf, initiating a retrograde pulse wave.

2 The cuffs inflate on the lower thigh.

3 The cuffs inflate on the upper thigh.

4 All three cuffs simultaneously deflate.

Cardiac rehabilitation

The goal of cardiac rehabilitation is to monitor and improve the patient's cardiovascular status, thereby reversing the cardiac disease process and improving the patient's overall physical condition and quality of life. In addition to exercise, cardiac rehabilitation includes:

■ managing stress
■ controlling diet, nutrition, and weight
■ reducing risk factors.

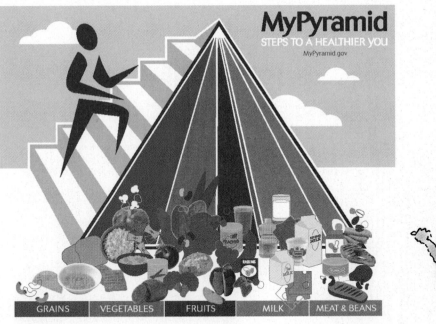

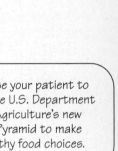

Advise your patient to use the U.S. Department of Agriculture's new MyPyramid to make healthy food choices.

Treatments for cardiomyopathy

You know it's bad when I need a VAD.

VAD

A ventricular assist device (VAD) is an implantable device that consists of a blood pump, cannulas, and a pneumatic or electrical drive console. The pump is synchronized to the patient's ECG and functions as the heart's ventricle. It decreases the heart's workload while increasing cardiac output.

Left VAD

A completely implanted left VAD is shown here.

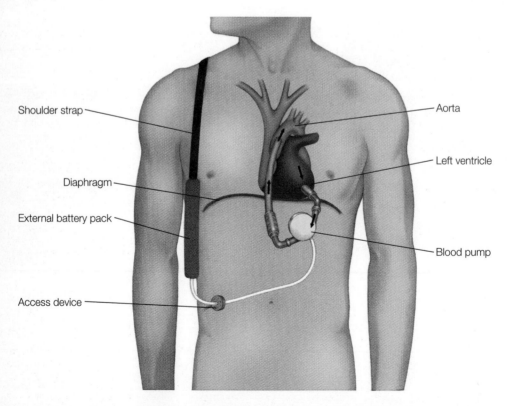

Shoulder strap

Diaphragm

External battery pack

Access device

Aorta

Left ventricle

Blood pump

Pump options

VADs are available as continuous flow or pulsatile pumps. A continuous flow pump fills continuously and returns blood to the aorta at a constant rate. A pulsatile pump may work in one of two ways:

 It may fill during systole and pump blood into the aorta during diastole.

 It may pump regardless of the patient's cardiac cycle.

Potential complications

Despite the use of anticoagulants, a VAD may cause thrombi formation, leading to pulmonary embolism or stroke. Other complications may include heart failure, bleeding, cardiac tamponade, or infection.

A closer look at VADs

There are three types of VADs.

1 A right VAD provides pulmonary support by diverting blood from the failing right ventricle to the VAD, which then pumps the blood to the pulmonary circulation via the VAD connection to the left pulmonary artery.

2 With a left VAD, blood flows from the left ventricle to the VAD, which then pumps blood back to the body via the VAD connection to the aorta.

3 When a right and left VAD are used, it's referred to as a *biventricular VAD (BiVAD)*.

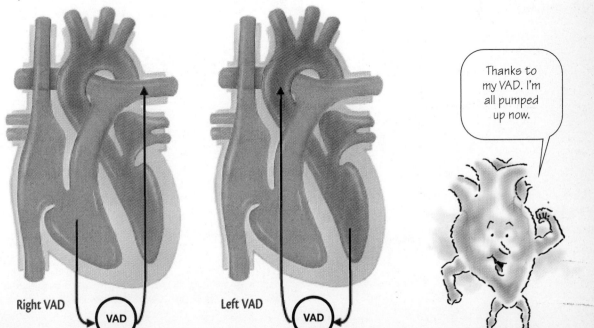

Right VAD   VAD

Left VAD   VAD

Thanks to my VAD. I'm all pumped up now.

Heart transplantation

In heart transplantation, a patient's failing heart is replaced with a donor heart. Used only to treat end-stage cardiac disease in patients who have poor quality of life and aren't expected to survive for more than 6 to 12 months, heart transplantation doesn't provide a cure.

Patients who receive donor hearts must be treated for rejection with monoclonal antibodies and potent immunosuppressants that can increase the risk of life-threatening infection.

> Before the donor's heart can be transplanted, the patient's failing heart is removed from his chest.

photo op

Heart transplantation surgery

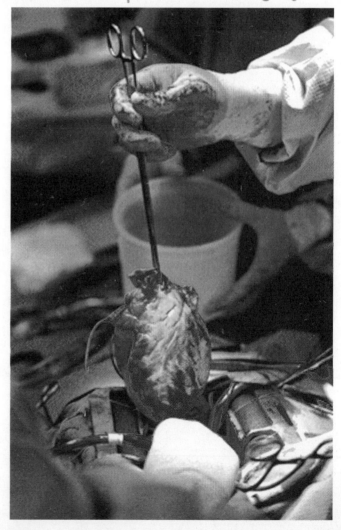

Heart to heart

The donor's heart

The donor's heart is removed after the surgeon cuts along these dissection lines.

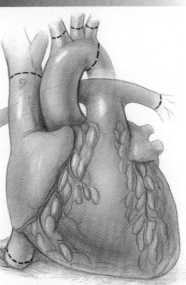

Anterior view

The recipient's heart

Before it can be removed, the recipient's heart is resected along these lines.

The transplanted heart

The transplanted heart is sutured.

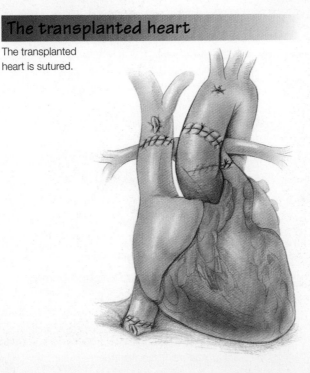

Valve treatments

Valve treatments are used to prevent heart failure in patients with valvular stenosis or insufficiency accompanied by severe, unmanageable symptoms. Depending on your patient's condition, he may undergo one of three types of valve surgery. When valve surgery isn't an option, percutaneous balloon valvuloplasty is used to enlarge the orifice of a stenotic heart valve, improving valvular function.

Valve replacement

In valve replacement, the natural heart valve is excised and a prosthetic valve is sutured in place.

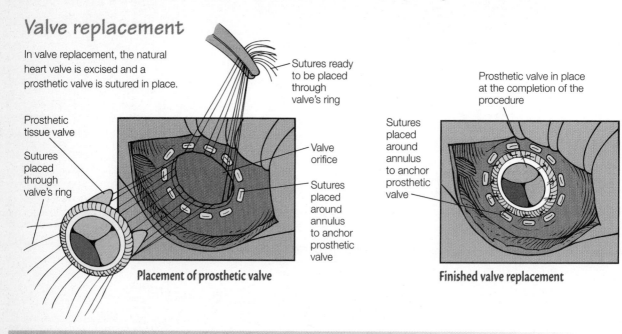

Prosthetic tissue valve

Sutures placed through valve's ring

Sutures ready to be placed through valve's ring

Valve orifice

Sutures placed around annulus to anchor prosthetic valve

Placement of prosthetic valve

Prosthetic valve in place at the completion of the procedure

Sutures placed around annulus to anchor prosthetic valve

Finished valve replacement

Types of replacement valves

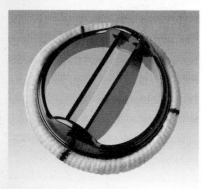

**Bileaflet valve
(St. Jude, mechanical)**

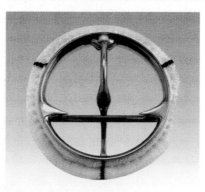

**Tilting-disk valve
(Medtronic-Hall, mechanical)**

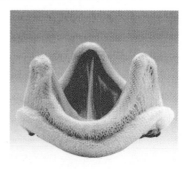

**Porcine heterograft valve
(Carpentier-Edwards, tissue)**

Valve leaflet resection and repair

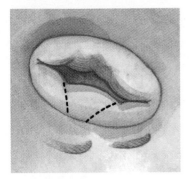

The section between the dashed lines is excised.

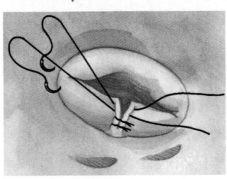

The edges are approximated and sutured.

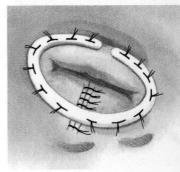

The repair is finished off with an annuloplasty ring.

Commissurotomy

In commissurotomy, the thickened leaflets are surgically separated.

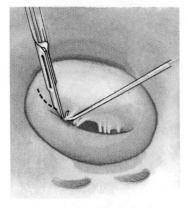

Commissurotomy of mitral valve

Percutaneous balloon valvuloplasty

During valvuloplasty, a surgeon inserts a small balloon catheter through the skin at the femoral vein and advances it until it reaches the affected valve. The balloon is then inflated, forcing the valve opening to widen.

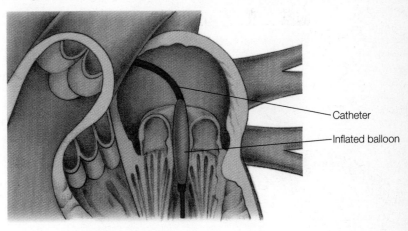

Catheter

Inflated balloon

Vascular repair

Vascular repair is a surgical option used to fix damaged or diseased vessels. Types of vascular repair include aortic aneurysm resection, bypass grafting, embolectomy, and vena caval filter insertion.

Aortic aneurysm resection

Aortic aneurysm resection involves removing an aneurysmal segment of the aorta. The surgeon first makes an incision to expose the aneurysm site. He then clamps the aorta, resects the aneurysm, and repairs the damaged portion of the aorta by sewing a prosthetic graft into place.

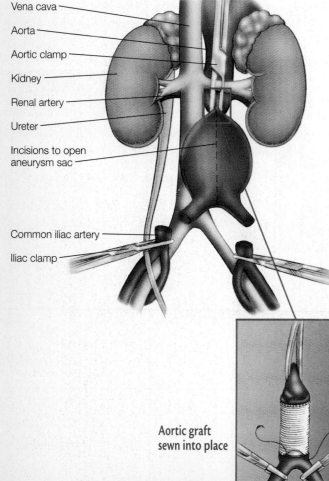

Vena cava

Aorta

Aortic clamp

Kidney

Renal artery

Ureter

Incisions to open aneurysm sac

Common iliac artery

Iliac clamp

Aortic graft sewn into place

Bypass grafting

Bypass grafting serves to bypass an arterial obstruction resulting from arteriosclerosis. After exposing the affected artery, the surgeon anastomoses a synthetic or autogenous graft to divert blood flow around the occluded arterial segment. This illustration shows a femoropopliteal bypass.

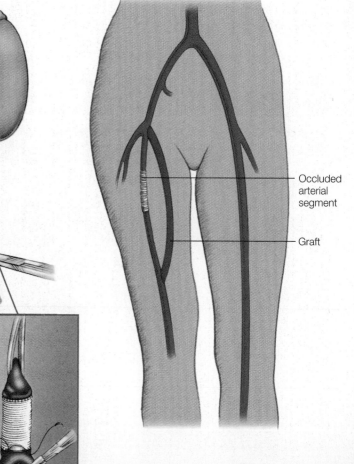

Occluded arterial segment

Graft

Embolectomy

To remove an embolism from an artery, a surgeon may perform an embolectomy by inserting a balloon-tipped indwelling catheter in the artery and passing it through the embolus (as shown below left). He then inflates the balloon and withdraws the catheter to remove the occlusion (as shown below right).

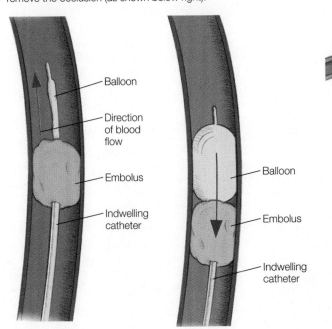

Balloon

Direction of blood flow

Embolus

Indwelling catheter

Balloon

Embolus

Indwelling catheter

Vena caval filter insertion

A vena caval filter, or umbrella, traps emboli in the vena cava, preventing them from reaching the pulmonary vessels but allowing venous blood flow.

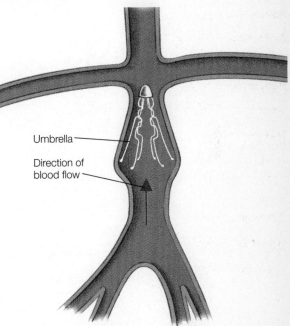

Umbrella

Direction of blood flow

Treatments for arrhythmias

Temporary pacing

Temporary pacing is used in arrhythmic emergencies, such as bradycardia and tachyarrhythmias, or other conduction system disturbances. Temporary pacemakers contain external, battery-powered pulse generators and a lead or electrode system.

Transcutaneous electrode placement

For a noninvasive temporary pacemaker, the two pacing electrodes are placed at heart level on the patient's chest and back, as shown. This type of pacemaker can be quickly applied in an emergency but is uncomfortable for the patient.

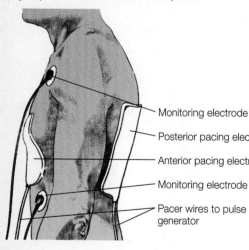

Monitoring electrode

Posterior pacing electrode

Anterior pacing electrode

Monitoring electrode

Pacer wires to pulse generator

Bradycardia algorithm

Bradycardia
Heart rate < 60 beats/minute and inadequate for clinical condition

- Maintain patent airway; assist breathing as needed.
- Give oxygen.
- Monitor ECG (identify rhythm), blood pressure, oximetry.
- Establish I.V. access.

Signs or symptoms of poor perfusion caused by bradycardia?
(acute altered mental status, ongoing chest pain,
hypotension, or other signs of shock)

ADEQUATE PERFUSION	**POOR PERFUSION**

Observe and monitor.

- Prepare for transcutaneous pacing; use without delay for high-degree block (type II second-degree block or third-degree AV block).
- Consider atropine while awaiting pacer. May repeat to a total dose of 3 mg. If ineffective, begin pacing.
- Consider epinephrine or dopamine infusion while awaiting pacer or if pacing is ineffective.

- Prepare for transvenous pacing.
- Treat contributing causes.
- Consider expert consultation.

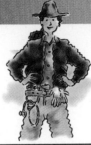

Come equipped

Transvenous pulse generator

Sense meter registers every time the patient's heart beats.

Pace meter registers every pacing stimulus delivered to the heart.

Rate control sets the heart rate below which the pacemaker takes over.

Sensitivity control adjusts pacemaker sensitivity to the patient's heart rate. When the dial is set on ASYNC, the pacemaker delivers a set rate regardless of the patient's intrinsic rate.

Output control determines the number of milliamps of electricity sent to the heart.

On-off switch activates the pulse generator.

Battery compartment

Connector attaches the pacing wires to the pulse generator.

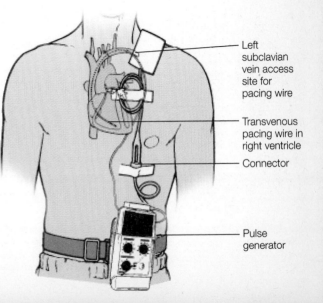

Temporary transvenous pacemaker

Transvenous pacing provides a more reliable pacing beat. This type of pacing is more comfortable for the patient because the pacing wire is inserted in the heart via a major vein.

Left subclavian vein access site for pacing wire

Transvenous pacing wire in right ventricle

Connector

Pulse generator

Permanent pacing

A permanent pacemaker is a self-contained device that's surgically implanted in a pocket under the patient's skin. Pacemakers treat persistent bradyarrhythmias, complete heart block, congenital or degenerative heart diseases, Stokes-Adams syndrome, Wolff-Parkinson-White syndrome, and sick sinus syndrome. Pacing electrodes can be placed in the atria, the ventricles, or both chambers (atrioventricular sequential or dual chamber). Biventricular pacemakers also are available for cardiac resynchronization therapy in patients with heart failure.

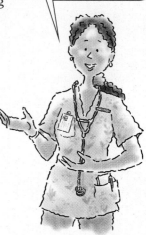

Permanent pacemakers allow the patient's heart to beat on its own but keep the heartbeat from falling below a preset rate.

Pacemaker lead enters external jugular vein

Pacemaker lead tunneled subcutaneously between pacemaker and external jugular vein

Generator placed beneath skin in pectoral region

Tip of wire (electrode) lodged in apex of right ventricle

Biventricular pacemaker

A biventricular pacemaker utilizes three leads: one to pace the right atrium, one to pace the right ventricle, and one to pace the left ventricle. The left ventricular lead is placed in the coronary sinus. Both ventricles are paced at the same time, causing them to contract simultaneously, improving cardiac output.

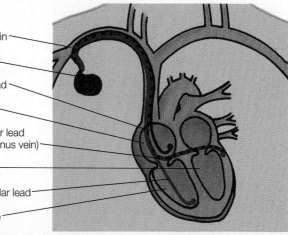

Subclavian vein

Generator

Right atrial lead

Right atrium

Left ventricular lead (in coronary sinus vein)

Left ventricle

Right ventricular lead

Right ventricle

Understanding pacemaker codes

A   **S**   **P**

First letter

Identifies heart chambers that are paced:
V = Ventricle
A = Atrium
D = Dual (ventricle and atrium)
O = None

Second letter

Signifies the heart chamber where the pacemaker senses the intrinsic activity:
V = Ventricle
A = Atrium
D = Dual
O = None

Third letter

Shows the pacemaker's response to the intrinsic electrical activity it senses in the atrium or ventricle:
T = Triggers pacing
I = Inhibits pacing
D = Dual (can be triggered or inhibited depending on the mode and where intrinsic activity occurs)
O = None (the pacemaker doesn't change its mode in response to sensed activity)

memory board

The letters of the pacemaker code help you to understand what the pacemaker is doing. To remember this important **ASP**ect of pacemaker coding, think of Cleopatra's **ASP**:
Assisted heart chamber
Sensed heart chamber
Pacemaker response to intrinsic activity it sensed.

> Asp-ed and answered. The most common pacing codes are VVI (single-chamber pacing) and DDD (dual-chamber pacing).

Pacemaker spikes

Pacemaker impulses—the stimuli that travel from the pacemaker to the heart—are visible on the patient's ECG tracing as spikes. Large or small, pacemaker spikes appear above or below the isoelectric line. This example shows an atrial and a ventricular pacemaker spike.

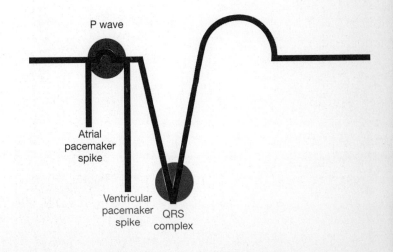

P wave

Atrial pacemaker spike

Ventricular pacemaker spike

QRS complex

Synchronized cardioversion

Synchronized cardioversion, also called *synchronized countershock*, is an elective or emergency procedure used to correct tachyarrhythmias. An electric current is delivered to the heart at a much lower energy level than used in defibrillation. The shock is synchronized to the peak R wave, causing immediate depolarization, interrupting reentry circuits and allowing the SA node to resume control.

If the patient's cardiac rhythm changes to ventricular fibrillation during cardioversion, the modes can be switched from "synchronized" to "defibrillate" and the patient can be defibrillated immediately after the machine is recharged. The sync mode must be reset on the defibrillator after each synchronized cardioversion (most defibrillators automatically reset to an unsynchronized mode).

Choosing the correct cardioversion energy level

When choosing an energy level for cardioversion, try the lowest energy level first. If the arrhythmia isn't corrected, repeat the procedure using the next energy level until the arrhythmia is corrected or until you reach the highest energy level.

Monophasic energy doses for cardioversion

For unstable monomorphic ventricular tachycardia with a pulse	For unstable paroxysmal supraventricular tachycardia	For unstable atrial fibrillation with rapid ventricular response	For unstable atrial flutter with rapid ventricular response
100 joules	50 joules	100 joules	50 joules
200 joules	100 joules	200 joules	100 joules
300 joules	200 joules	300 joules	200 joules
360 joules	300 joules	360 joules	300 joules
	360 joules		360 joules

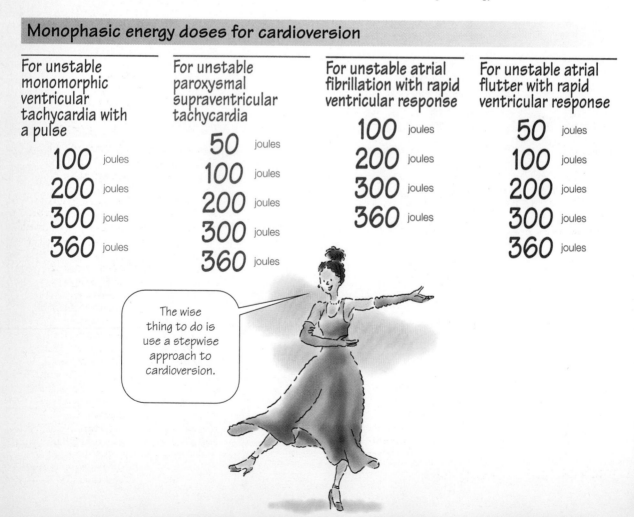

The wise thing to do is use a stepwise approach to cardioversion.

Tachycardia algorithm

1 **Tachycardia with pulses**

2
- Assess and support ABCs as needed.
- Give oxygen.
- Monitor ECG (identify rhythm), blood pressure, oximetry.
- Identify and treat reversible causes.

Symptoms persist

3
Is patient stable?
Unstable signs include altered mental status, ongoing chest pain, hypotension or other signs of shock.

Unstable

4
Perform immediate synchronized cardioversion.
- Establish I.V. access and give sedation if patient is conscious; do not delay cardioversion.
- Consider expert consultation.
- If pulseless arrest develops, see pulseless arrest algorithm, page 224.

Stable

5
- Establish I.V. access.
- Obtain 12-lead ECG (when available) or rhythm strip.
Is QRS narrow?

Narrow (<0.12 sec)

6
Narrow QRS*
Is rhythm regular?

Wide (≥0.12 sec)

12
Wide QRS*
Is rhythm regular?
Expert consultation advised.

Regular

7
- Attempt vagal maneuvers.
- Give adenosine 6 mg rapid I.V. push. If no conversion, give 12 mg rapid I.V. push; may repeat 12-mg dose once.

Irregular

11
Irregular Narrow-Complex Tachycardia
Probable atrial fibrillation or possible atrial flutter or multifocal atrial tachycardia
- Consider expert consultation.
- Control rate (diltiazem, beta blockers; use beta blockers with caution in pulmonary disease or heart failure).

Regular

13
If ventricular tachycardia or uncertain rhythm
- Amiodarone 150 mg I.V. over 10 min. Repeat as needed to maximum dosage of 2.2 g/24 hours.
- Prepare for elective synchronized cardioversion.
If SVT with aberrancy
- Give adenosine (go to box 7).

Irregular

14
If atrial fibrillation with aberrancy
- See Irregular Narrow-Complex Tachycardia (box 11).
If pre-excited atrial fibrillation (AF + WPW)
- Expert consultation advised.
- Avoid AV nodal blocking agents (adenosine, digoxin, diltiazem, verapamil).
- Consider antiarrhythmics (amiodarone 150 mg I.V. over 10 min).
If recurrent polymorphic VT
- Seek expert consultation.
If torsades de pointes
- Give magnesium (load with 1 to 2 g over 5 to 60 min, then infusion).

8
Does rhythm convert?
Note: Consider expert consultation.

Converts

9
If rhythm converts, probably reentry supraventricular tachycardia (SVT)
- Observe for recurrence.
- Treat recurrence with adenosine or longer-acting AV nodal blocking agents (such as diltiazem or beta blockers).

Does not convert

10
If rhythm does NOT convert, possible atrial flutter, ectopic atrial tachycardia, or junctional tachycardia
- Control rate (diltiazem, beta blockers; use beta blockers with caution in pulmonary disease or heart failure).
- Treat underlying cause.
- Consider expert consultation.

* Note: If patient becomes unstable, go to box 4.

Implantable cardioverter defibrillation

Implantable cardioverter defibrillators (ICDs) are used for antiarrhythmic pacing, cardioversion, and defibrillation. Some defibrillators have the ability to pace the atrium and the ventricle, and some can perform biventricular pacing. A lead or leads are placed transvenously in the endocardium of the appropriate chambers. The lead connects to a generator box implanted in the right or left upper chest near the clavicle.

> An ICD typically consists of a programmable pulse generator and an electrode. It detects ventricular bradyarrhythmias and tachyarrhythmias and responds with appropriate therapies.

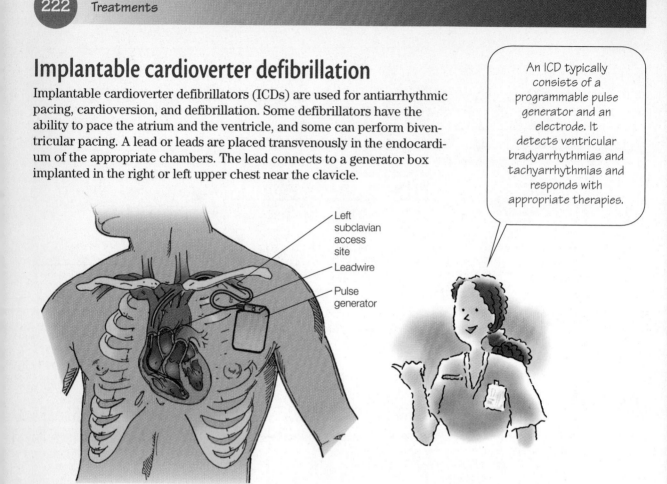

Left subclavian access site

Leadwire

Pulse generator

Types of ICD therapies

ICDs can deliver a range of therapies depending on the arrhythmia that's detected and how the device is programmed. These include antitachycardia pacing, cardioversion, defibrillation, and bradycardia pacing.

Therapy	What it does
Antitachycardia pacing	A series of small, rapid, electrical pacing pulses are used to interrupt ventricular tachycardia (VT) and return the heart to its normal rhythm.
Cardioversion	A low- or high-energy shock (up to 35 joules) is timed to the R wave to terminate VT and return the heart to its normal rhythm.
Defibrillation	A high-energy shock (up to 35 joules) to the heart is used to terminate ventricular fibrillation and return the heart to its normal rhythm.
Bradycardia pacing	Electrical pacing pulses are used when the heart's natural electrical signals are too slow. Most ICD systems can pace one chamber (VVI pacing) of the heart at a preset rate. Some systems will sense and pace both chambers (DDD pacing).

Radiofrequency ablation

Radiofrequency ablation is used to treat arrhythmias in patients who don't respond to antiarrhythmic drugs or cardioversion. During the procedure, a special catheter is inserted in a vein and advanced to the heart. After the source of the arrhythmia is identified, radiofrequency energy destroys the abnormal electrical impulses or conduction pathway. The tissue that's destroyed can no longer conduct electrical impulses.

Types of ablation

AV node ablation

If a rapid arrhythmia originates above the AV node, the AV node may be destroyed to block impulses from reaching the ventricles. A pacemaker may then be required to stimulate the ventricles.

The radiofrequency ablation catheter is directed to the AV node.

Pulmonary vein ablation

If a pulmonary vein is the source of the arrhythmia, such as in atrial fibrillation, radiofrequency energy is used to destroy the tissue in the area of the atrium that connects to the pulmonary vein. The scar that forms blocks impulses from firing within the pulmonary vein, preventing the arrhythmia.

The radiofrequency catheter is directed to the base of the pulmonary vein.

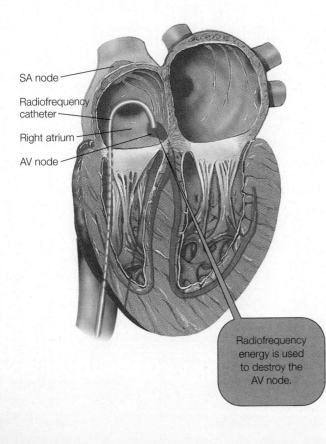

SA node
Radiofrequency catheter
Right atrium
AV node

Radiofrequency energy is used to destroy the AV node.

Pulmonary vein

SA node
Radiofrequency catheter

Radiofrequency energy is used to destroy the tissue where the atrium connects to the pulmonary vein.

Pulseless arrest algorithm

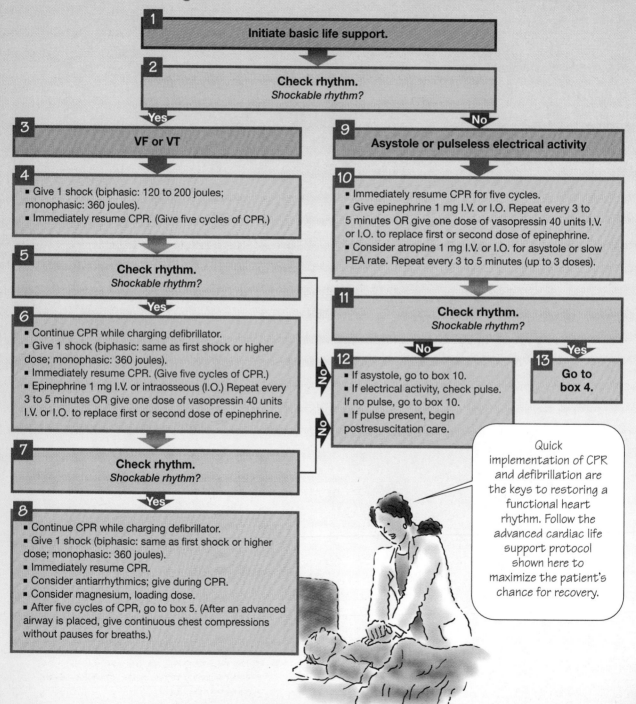

1 Initiate basic life support.

2 Check rhythm.
Shockable rhythm?

Yes → **3** VF or VT

No → **9** Asystole or pulseless electrical activity

4
- Give 1 shock (biphasic: 120 to 200 joules; monophasic: 360 joules).
- Immediately resume CPR. (Give five cycles of CPR.)

5 Check rhythm.
Shockable rhythm?

Yes → **6**
- Continue CPR while charging defibrillator.
- Give 1 shock (biphasic: same as first shock or higher dose; monophasic: 360 joules).
- Immediately resume CPR. (Give five cycles of CPR.)
- Epinephrine 1 mg I.V. or intraosseous (I.O.) Repeat every 3 to 5 minutes OR give one dose of vasopressin 40 units I.V. or I.O. to replace first or second dose of epinephrine.

7 Check rhythm.
Shockable rhythm?

Yes → **8**
- Continue CPR while charging defibrillator.
- Give 1 shock (biphasic: same as first shock or higher dose; monophasic: 360 joules).
- Immediately resume CPR.
- Consider antiarrhythmics; give during CPR.
- Consider magnesium, loading dose.
- After five cycles of CPR, go to box 5. (After an advanced airway is placed, give continuous chest compressions without pauses for breaths.)

10
- Immediately resume CPR for five cycles.
- Give epinephrine 1 mg I.V. or I.O. Repeat every 3 to 5 minutes OR give one dose of vasopressin 40 units I.V. or I.O. to replace first or second dose of epinephrine.
- Consider atropine 1 mg I.V. or I.O. for asystole or slow PEA rate. Repeat every 3 to 5 minutes (up to 3 doses).

11 Check rhythm.
Shockable rhythm?

No → **12**
- If asystole, go to box 10.
- If electrical activity, check pulse. If no pulse, go to box 10.
- If pulse present, begin postresuscitation care.

Yes → **13** Go to box 4.

No

No

> Quick implementation of CPR and defibrillation are the keys to restoring a functional heart rhythm. Follow the advanced cardiac life support protocol shown here to maximize the patient's chance for recovery.

Cardiopulmonary resuscitation

Effective CPR requires compressions that are hard, fast, accurately placed, and allow complete chest recoil. If a second rescuer arrives, chest compressions should be continuous and ventilation should be provided at 8 to 10 breaths per minute during compressions.

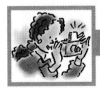

photo op

Performing one-person CPR

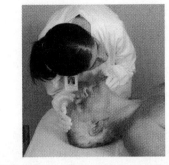

After initiating the emergency response team or calling for a defibrillator when a patient is unresponsive, position the patient supine on a hard surface and open the airway. Then check for adequate breathing for 10 seconds.

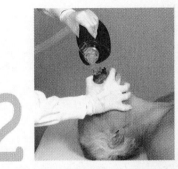

Perform ventilation with 2 breaths that make the chest rise, at 1 second per breath. If ineffective, reposition the airway and retry.

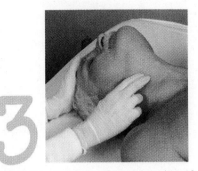

Palpate the carotid pulse for no more than 10 seconds. Unless a definite pulse is felt, initiate chest compressions.

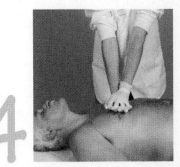

Place hands one on top of the other on the lower half of the sternum between the nipples, with elbows locked. Compress the chest 1½″ to 2″ (or one-third the depth of the chest) at a rate of 100 compressions per minute, keeping your hands on the chest. Allow equal time for compression and full chest recoil. Continue for 30 compressions, then give 2 ventilations and resume compressions quickly for five cycles (2 minutes) before rechecking the pulse.

Defibrillation

In defibrillation, electrode paddles direct an electric current through the patient's heart, causing the myocardium to depolarize, which in turn encourages the SA node to resume control of the heart's electrical activity. Because some arrhythmias can cause death, the success of defibrillation depends on early recognition and intervention.

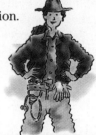

Placing the paddles

During defibrillation, place the paddles as shown. During cardiac surgery, smaller paddles may be placed directly on the myocardium.

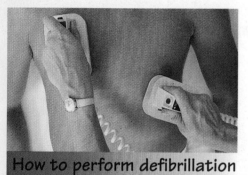

How to perform defibrillation

To perform external defibrillation on an adult, give one shock. The number of joules to give depends on the machine being used:
- monophasic — 360 joules
- biphasic — see manufacturer's instructions
- automated external defibrillator — preset by the machine.

If your patient doesn't have a pulse after defibrillation, quickly resume CPR for 2 minutes and then reattempt defibrillation.

Come equipped

The defibrillator

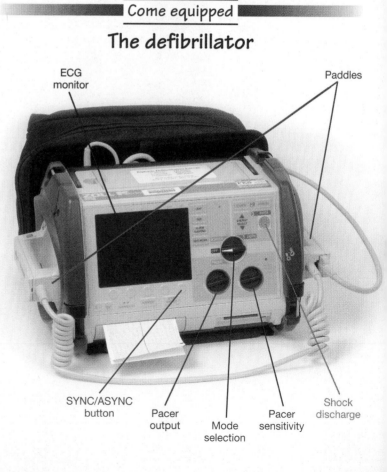

ECG monitor

Paddles

SYNC/ASYNC button

Pacer output

Mode selection

Pacer sensitivity

Shock discharge

Automated external defibrillation

An automated external defibrillator (AED) has a cardiac rhythm analysis system that interprets the patient's cardiac rhythm and gives the operator step-by-step directions on how to proceed. This device was designed to allow laypeople with CPR and AED training to initiate care in an emergency until medical staff arrive.

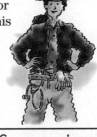

Come equipped

The AED

An AED has a "quick-look" feature that analyzes a patient's heart rhythm. This feature allows you to visualize the heart's rhythm by pushing a button after the electrodes are connected. Then the defibrillator audibly and visually prompts you to deliver a shock, if needed.

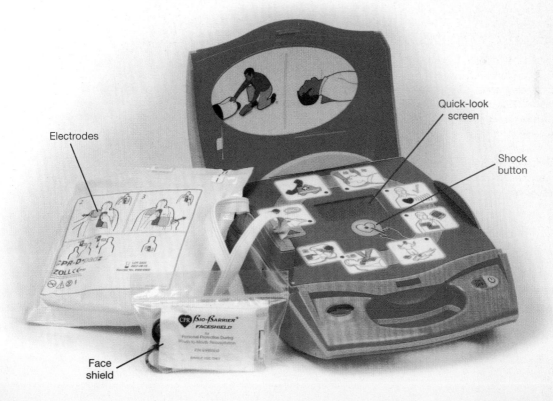

Electrodes

Quick-look screen

Shock button

Face shield

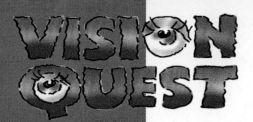

Matchmaker

Match the equipment in the pictures at right with the procedures for which they're used.

1.

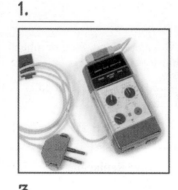

2.

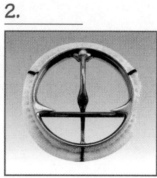

3.

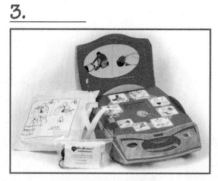

A. Temporary pacing

B. Automated external defibrillation

C. Valve replacement

Photo finish

Number these photos in the correct step-by-step order for performing CPR.

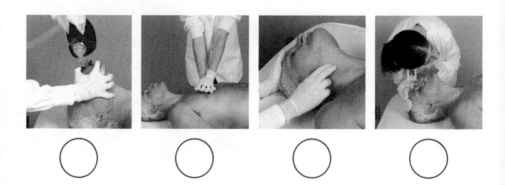

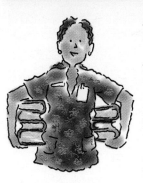

Anatomy & Physiology Made Incredibly Easy, 2nd ed. Philadelphia: Lippincott Williams & Wilkins, 2005.

Assessment Made Incredibly Easy, 3rd ed. Philadelphia: Lippincott Williams & Wilkins, 2005.

Bickley, L.S., and Szilagyi, P.G. *Bates' Guide to Physical Examination and History Taking*, 9th ed. Philadelphia: Lippincott Williams & Wilkins, 2006.

Cardiovascular Care Made Incredibly Easy, 3rd ed. Philadelphia: Lippincott Williams & Wilkins, 2005.

Darovic, G.O. *Handbook of Hemodynamic Monitoring*, 2nd ed. Philadelphia: W.B. Saunders Co., 2006.

Fink, A.M. "Endocarditis after Valve Replacement Surgery," *AJN* 106(2):40-51, February 2006.

Ignatavicius, D.D., and Workman, M.L. *Medical-Surgical Nursing: Critical Thinking for Collaborative Care*, 5th ed. Philadelphia: W.B. Saunders Co., 2006.

Kasper, D.L., et al., eds. *Harrison's Principles of Internal Medicine*, 16th ed. New York: McGraw-Hill Book Co., 2005.

Woods, S.L., et al. *Cardiac Nursing*, 5th ed. Philadelphia: Lippincott Williams & Wilkins, 2005.

Yoon, J.O. "Not Just an Aneurysm, but an Infected One: A Case Report and Literature," *Journal of Vascular Nursing* 24(1):2-8, March 2006.

Credits

Chapter 2

Interview, page 22. Smeltzer, S.C., and Bare, B.G. *Brunner and Suddarth's Textbook of Medical-Surgical Nursing*, 10th ed. Philadelphia: Lippincott Williams & Wilkins, 2003.

Pitting edema, page 40. From Bickley, L.S., and Szilagyi, P. *Bates' Guide to Physical Examination and History Taking*, 8th ed. Philadelphia: Lippincott Williams & Wilkins, 2003.

Chapter 3

Echocardiogram, page 62; Doppler of popliteal artery, page 72. Smeltzer, S.C., and Bare, B.G. *Brunner and Suddarth's Textbook of Medical-Surgical Nursing*, 10th ed. Philadelphia: Lippincott Williams & Wilkins, 2003.

MRI scanner, page 66. © 2006 JupiterImage.

MRI image, page 66; Angiograph of femoral artery and its branches, page 75. Dean, D., and Herbener, T. E. *Cross-Sectional Human Anatomy*. Baltimore: Lippincott Williams & Wilkins, 2000.

Cardiac blood pool imaging, pages 68 and 69. Images © Texas Heart Institute *www.texasheartinstitute.org.*

Thallium study image, page 71. Obtained from "My Physiology" learning resource, in *PenneyLibrary.com* by David G. Penney.

Measuring ankle-brachial index, page 73. Equipment is shown courtesy of D.E. Hokanson, Inc.

Chapter 6

Libman-Sacks and bacterial endocarditis, page 133; Viral myocarditis, page 136; Chronic constrictive pericarditis, page 138; Aortic stenosis, page 146; Pitting edema, page 154; Locations of aortic aneurysms, page 166. Rubin, E., and Farber, J.L. *Pathology*, 3rd ed. Philadelphia: Lippincott Williams & Wilkins, 1999.

Pulmonary hypertension, page 150. Cagle, P.T. *Color Atlas and Text of Pulmonary Pathology*. Philadelphia: Lippincott Williams & Wilkins, 2005.

Looking for edema, page 154. From Bickley, L.S., and Szilagyi, P. *Bates' Guide to Physical Examination and History Taking*, 8th ed. Philadelphia: Lippincott Williams & Wilkins, 2003.

Dissecting aneurysm, page 167. Cohen, B.J. *Medical Terminology*, 4th ed. Philadelphia: Lippincott Williams & Wilkins, 2003.

Arterial ulcer, page 168. Nettina, S.M. *Lippincott Manual of Nursing Practice*, 8th ed. Philadelphia: Lippincott Williams & Wilkins, 2005.

Chapter 7

Positioning for shock, page 181. Smeltzer, S.C., and Bare, B.G. *Brunner and Suddarth's Textbook of Medical-Surgical Nursing*, 10th ed. Philadelphia: Lippincott Williams & Wilkins, 2003.

MI and cardiac tamponade, page 182. Rubin, E., and Farber, J.L. *Pathology*, 3rd ed. Philadelphia: Lippincott Williams & Wilkins, 1999.

Chapter 8

Treating hypertension algorithm, page 192. U.S. Department of Health and Human Services, *The Seventh Report of the Joint National Committee on Prevention, Detection, Evaluation, and Treatment of High Blood Pressure* (NIH Publication No. 03-5233), December 2003.

Coronary artery bypass graft surgery, pages 196 and 197. Neil O. Hardy, Westpoint, Connecticut.

Vein graft for bypass suturing vein (CABG inset), page 197. © Barber/Custom Medical Stock Photo.

Open heart surgery bypass pump (in "Performing CABG surgery"), page 197. © SIUCustom Medical Stock Photo.

Understanding PTCA, page 202. Cohen, B.J. *Medical Terminology*, 4th ed. Philadelphia: Lippincott Williams & Wilkins, 2003.

Intravascular stents, page 203. Willis, M.C. *Medical Terminology: A Programmed Learning Approach to the Language of Health Care*. Baltimore: Lippincott Williams & Wilkins, 2002.

MyPyramid, page 207. Adapted from *www.MyPyramid.gov.*

Heart transplantation surgery, page 210. Becky Sell for The Post, an independent, student-run newspaper serving Ohio University.

Valve replacement, page 212; Permanent pacing, page 218; Implantable cardioverter-defibrillator, page 222; Placing defibrillator paddles, page 226. Smeltzer, S.C., and Bare, B.G. *Brunner and Suddarth's Textbook of Medical-Surgical Nursing*, 10th ed. Philadelphia: Lippincott Williams & Wilkins, 2003.

Bileaflet valve (SJM Regent Valve), page 212. Image provided courtesy of St. Jude Medical, Inc. All rights reserved.

Tilting-disk valve (Medtronic Hall Mitral Valve), pages 212 and 228. Copyright Medtronic, Inc. Used with permission.

Porcine valve (Aortic-model 2650), page 212. Edwards Lifesciences, Irvine, California.

Bradycardia algorithm, page 216. Reproduced with permission. *2005 American Heart Association Guidelines for Cardiopulmonary Resuscitation and Emergency Cardiovascular Care.* © 2005, American Heart Association.

Tachycardia algorithm, page 221. Reproduced with permission. *2005 American Heart Association Guidelines for Cardiopulmonary Resuscitation and Emergency Cardiovascular Care.* © 2005, American Heart Association.

Pulseless arrest algorithm, page 224. Reproduced with permission. *2005 American Heart Association Guidelines for Cardiopulmonary Resuscitation and Emergency Cardiovascular Care.* © 2005, American Heart Association.

We gratefully acknowledge Anatomical Chart Company and LifeART for the use of selected images.

Index